THE
ENDURANCE
TRAINING
DIET & COOKBOOK

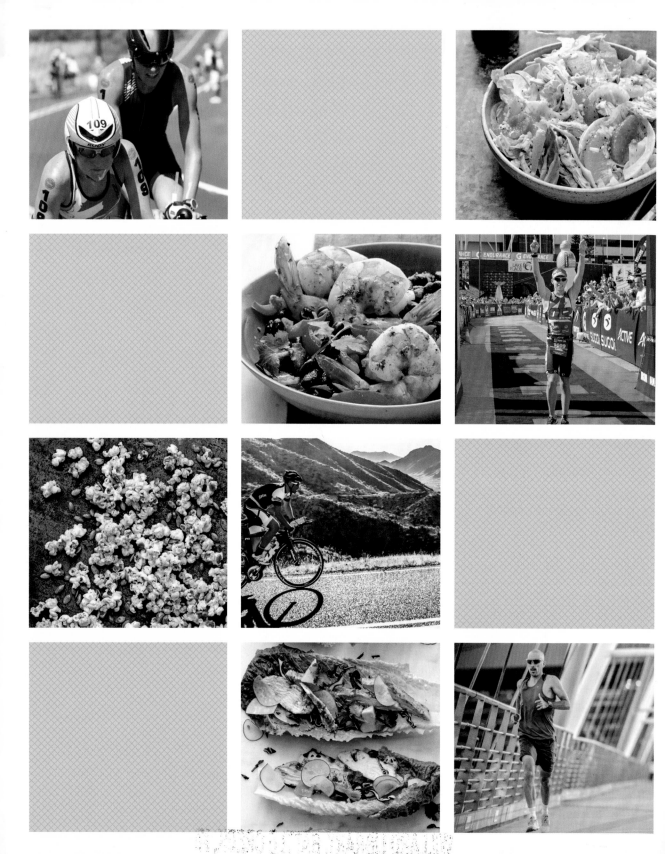

THE ENDURANCE TRAINING
DIET & COOKBOOK

The How, When, and What for
Fueling Runners and Triathletes
to Improve Performance

JESSE KROPELNICKI
FOUNDER OF THE CORE DIET™

Recipes by Shirley Fan, M.S., R.D.

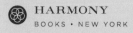
HARMONY
BOOKS • NEW YORK

Published in the United States by Harmony Books,
an imprint of the Crown Publishing Group, a division of
Penguin Random House LLC, New York.
crownpublishing.com

HARMONY BOOKS is a registered trademark, and the Circle
colophon is a trademark of Penguin Random House LLC.

All photographs by Andrew Purcell except as follows:
pages 2 (top left), 22, and 66, © 2016 by Charlie Abrahams
Photography; pages 2 (all except top left), 16–17, 53, and
86–87, © 2016 by Pedro Gomes; page 40, © 2016 by Fuse/
Corbis/Getty Images; pages 46–47 and 69, © 2016 by
ImageSource.com; pages 62 and 84, © 2016 by Chris Corbin;
page 80, © 2016 Masakazu Watanabe/Aflo/ Getty Images.

Library of Congress Cataloging-in-Publication Data
Names: Kropelnicki, Jesse, author.
Title: The endurance training diet & cookbook : the how,
    when, and what for fueling runners and triathletes to
    improve performance / Jesse Kropelnicki, Founder of the
    Core Diet.
Description: First edition. | New York : Harmony, [2017] |
    Includes index.
Identifiers: LCCN 2016008605| ISBN 9781101904602 (trade
    pbk. : alk. paper) | ISBN 9781101904619 (ebook)
Subjects: LCSH: Atheletes—Nutrition. | High-protein diet—
    Recipes. | High-fiber diet—Recipes. | LCGFT: Cookbooks.
Classification: LCC TX361.A8 K76 2017 | DDC 613.7/11—
    dc23 LC record available at https://lccn.loc.gov/
    2016008605

ISBN 978-1-101-90460-2
Ebook ISBN 978-1-101-90461-9

Printed in China
Book design by Kelley Galbreath
Jacket design by Kelley Galbreath
Jacket photographs by Andrew Purcell

10 9 8 7 6 5 4 3 2 1

First Edition

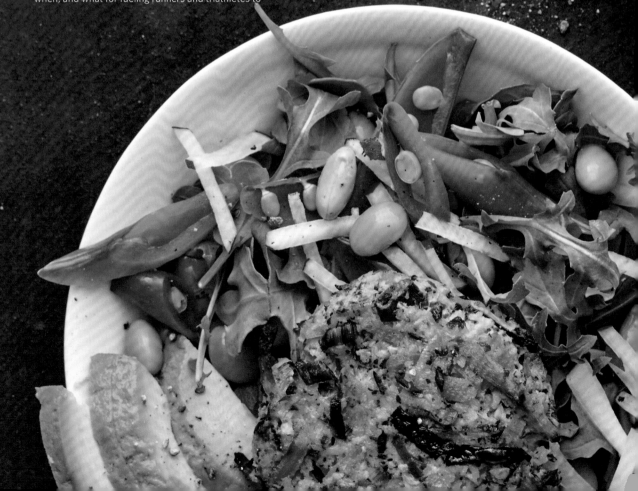

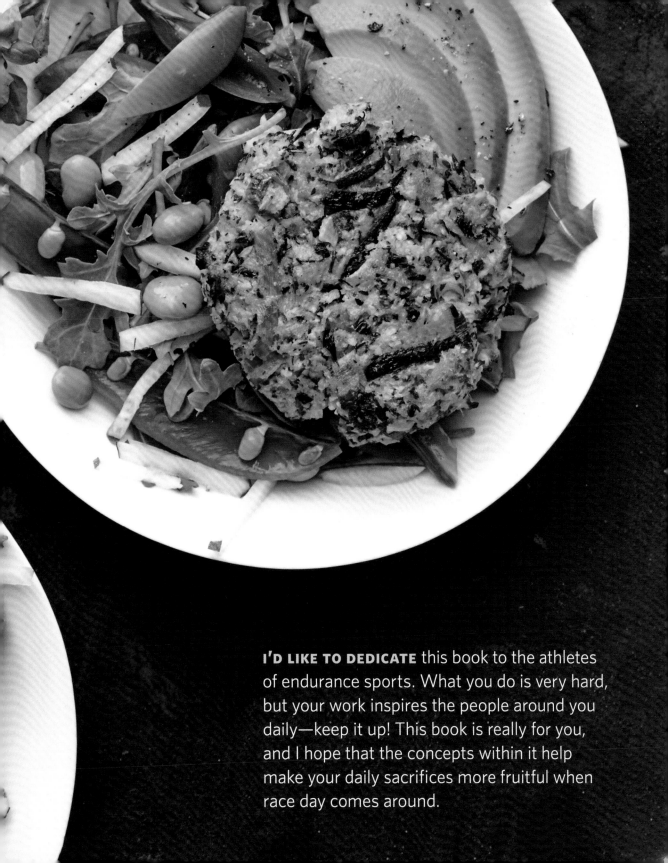

I'D LIKE TO DEDICATE this book to the athletes of endurance sports. What you do is very hard, but your work inspires the people around you daily—keep it up! This book is really for you, and I hope that the concepts within it help make your daily sacrifices more fruitful when race day comes around.

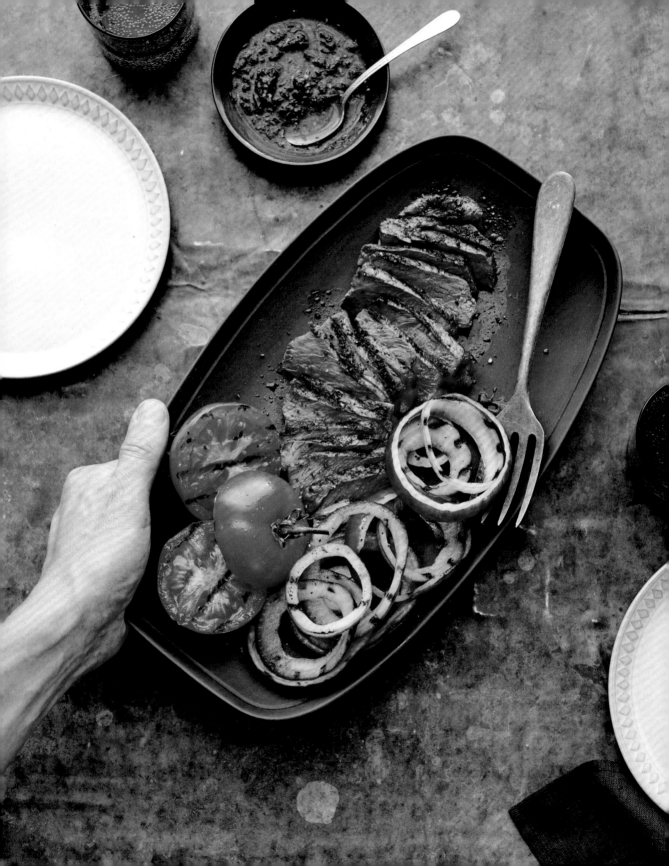

CONTENTS

INTRODUCTION

OVER THE COURSE OF EIGHTEEN YEARS of working with athletes of all types—including UFC fighters, dancers, and world-class triathletes—I've learned that there's much, much more to achieving the level of performance you're aiming for than fitness itself. By that I mean it's not just in the hard workouts balanced by the recovery days—the thoughtfully planned training strategies for fine-tuning an athlete's sport. The body needs food, since food is fuel, and as it turns out, the better a person eats, the better the body does its thing. It seems so simple, which is why it's astounding that what we eat affects our athletic performance so significantly, and yet very few athletes get it right.

Through my many years as a coach, I designed the Core Diet, my nutrition coaching company and eating philosophy, which isn't really a diet at all but rather a way of life for athletes. After seeing so many athletes spend significant amounts of time in training, making many sacrifices to put in the hours it takes to accomplish every workout, I noticed that very few would truly optimize their nutrition to support the training they were doing. This seemed like a massive opportunity and potential advantage to me, so I structured sports-nutrition concepts into an easy-to-understand set of tenants and began working with endurance athletes all over the world on their nutrition. Sure enough, my athletes began to reach higher levels of performance, breaking through time barriers and recovering faster than ever after racing events. My approach ended up being so successful with

the athletes I was working with that I trained a staff of registered dietitians to employ these concepts for all athletes, elite or not. Today, I coach more than a dozen professional IRONMAN athletes, as well as train coaches and dietitians around the world on the exact nutrition principles that are outlined in this book.

I've always been attuned to health, thanks to my upbringing. Like many children of the 1980s, I have a mother who was a naturalist interested in health and the use of homeopathic approaches with her own and our family's nutrition. She opted for supplemental vitamins and minerals instead of antibiotics or traditional medicines whenever possible. I can remember visiting the local health food store, which emanated a smell of sprouts and other earthy things, on a regular basis, looking up at the shelves of various supplements and thinking that there must be some magic in this stuff! These types of experiences ended up engraining an interest in nutrition and a focus on natural approaches in me. And I've always wanted to figure out that magic, though I knew pretty quickly that the answers probably couldn't be found in a bottle.

Later, as I focused on fitness, I began to think about finding a better way to fuel the body both in between training sessions and during. In 1997, I sat in a dorm room as a freshman in college, uninterested in the party scene and instead deeply passionate about weight lifting and civil engineering, my chosen major. At that time, I was working at a friend's supplement shop in

Boston, learning about various powders and pills, and talking with customers. There was even a three year period during which I tracked my macronutrient intake—proteins, carbohydrates, and fats—every single day. Yes, that's right, I can tell you exactly what I ate on June 3, 1998 (engineering was a good field for me). As crazy as it might sound, it was an amazing exercise that taught me how various food combinations can influence body composition and performance both in the gym and outside of the gym. During that time, although I was mostly lifting weights and looking to gain muscle mass, I raced in one sprint triathlon (in 1997) and had the bug to do more at some point. But I knew that the bulk that I'd been building over the past three or four years would hinder me in triathlon racing. In 2000, at a body weight of 205 pounds (up from 150 freshman year), I was ready to make changes to my nutrition program to better match my physique to the endurance sport's lean and slim look. I knew if I wanted to become a faster triathlete, I needed to get rid of muscle that may not be needed for the sport. In fact, I had about 45 pounds of unwanted muscle mass—that extra weight would definitely slow me down! Over the next five years, I slowly reduced this muscle by careful macronutrient manipulation, eventually getting down to a race weight of 158 pounds.

Through the process of manipulating my own body composition, I learned a tremendous amount about how the human body adapts to how you feed it, and how that intake dovetails with the way the body adjusts to your training load. I knew that there was a way to feed the body both in and out of training to help it do a lot of things: recover from training sessions, enhance immunity, promote health, and remove nutrition limiters during competition. These are the things that became the Core Diet, and I've now compiled all of these concepts in this book.

The Endurance Training Diet and Cookbook is two books in one. It starts out with a manual with lots of details regarding nutrition as it pertains to training and racing. Actually, I begin by walking through the basic tenets of a healthy diet and lifestyle, which is the foundation that all of us need to strive for in our day-to-day lives. And then I drill down into how nutrition can be a precise tool for getting your body into the best shape, increasing or decreasing muscle mass according to your needs, and supporting you as you maintain an intense level of physical exertion.

The second part of the book is recipes, all of which abide by my nutrition philosophy and can help you practically enact the tenets laid out in the first part of the book. Being an endurance athlete doesn't mean you're relegated to eating tons of breads, pastas, and grains. You'll find in the recipes so much color and variety—lots of vegetables, all sorts of proteins from fish to meats to eggs, and even a few all-natural desserts. Although I'm a proponent of consuming store-bought sports drinks, bars, and gels (only in appropriate windows), I also think you can make some of your own with great success, and so you'll find recipes for those as well. This is real food, made with whole foods, and every bit of it supports a healthy, active lifestyle.

I hope that you find *The Endurance Training Diet and Cookbook* interesting, informative, and, above all, useful. And I hope that you're able to break new ground in your training for better, faster—and more fun—racing.

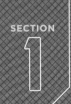

NUTR

RITION

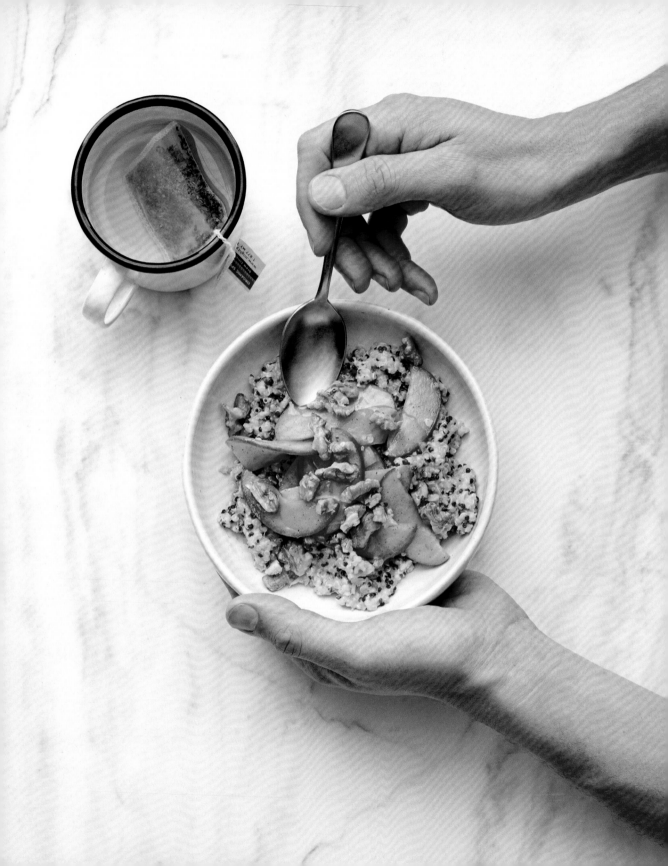

1

EAT WELL
FOR YOUR BEST
PERFORMANCE

DO YOU WANT TO GET AN EDGE in your half marathon, marathon, triathlon, and/or IRONMAN racing? So many athletes are striving to gain a margin of increased performance that allows them to reach their goals, but carefully crafting a workout schedule alone won't cut it—fueling properly is the key! Through the nutrition company I founded, I have worked with thousands of athletes and can tell you that the longer the race distance becomes, the more nutrition can actually limit results. I'd bet that most athletes who are unhappy with their race performances in races longer than 3 hours had inadequate nutrition as their primary limiter. People are learning the hard way that diet is more important than ever. To me, this is a sad fact, since it is so easy to address. I never like to see athletes who have made sacrifices in training, taking time away from their families and friends, have nutrition deficits be what holds them back on race day.

One big reason why improving your diet as it pertains to training and racing positively affects performance is that your body is better positioned to absorb training loads and handle additional stresses. The athlete who can apply and absorb the most training stress over the long haul makes the most progress. Good nutrition, day to day, in what and when you eat will help your body handle the increasing stressors of training so that on race day you'll be stronger than ever. The beginner athlete will benefit from learning the proper fundamentals right at the start, which sets the ideal nutritional stage for performance. Professional or elite athletes can use nutrition to gain that much-needed, extremely valuable 1% improvement—a seemingly small margin that can be the only thing keeping them from winning. So often I see athletes pushing for that margin with harder, longer training sessions, which tax the body immensely. But sometimes, simple dietary changes can help someone achieve that 1% without physical cost, and instead with an improved state of being that comes with eating well and recovering well. I recently worked with one top-level professional triathlete on race fueling, aiming to manage her body composition properly throughout the year, while also understanding her sweat rates and her specific sodium and fluid needs. A big part of the process was simply practicing good nutrition more intensely. She went from barely finishing her races to outstanding performance at the world championship in just 6 months! If that's not proof of how proper nutrition can help you, I'm not sure what is.

A HEALTHY LIFESTYLE AND OPTIMIZATION PHASES

The Endurance Training Diet and Cookbook promotes the philosophy that athletes should follow and maintain a lifestyle of healthy eating all of the time, and then augment their diets during training and racing seasons to support the vigorous work that they put their bodies through. The principles here are significant to the optimization of an athlete's body composition and will affect his or her performance, both directly and indirectly. But, much more important, these principles lead to healthier day-to-day living and well-being, as the foods I encourage you to eat will give you more energy and cause you to feel better in general.

A HEALTHY LIFESTYLE

Most athletes know that while a training program is necessary to prepare for any endurance race— gradually building up stamina and strength in order to finish strong on race day—having a base of fitness is also essential. Your marathon plan, for example, may list a run of 6 miles on day one, but it's far, far better if that isn't your first run of that distance! The body needs time to develop aptitude for such an activity, and so the months before that 6-mile run should include many runs of varying lengths, including a few 6-milers.

When it comes to nutrition, you should treat your body the same way. Totally changing your diet right as you begin training could result in some uncomfortable transitions (such as tummy aches or other unsettled digestive results). But, more important, you need a

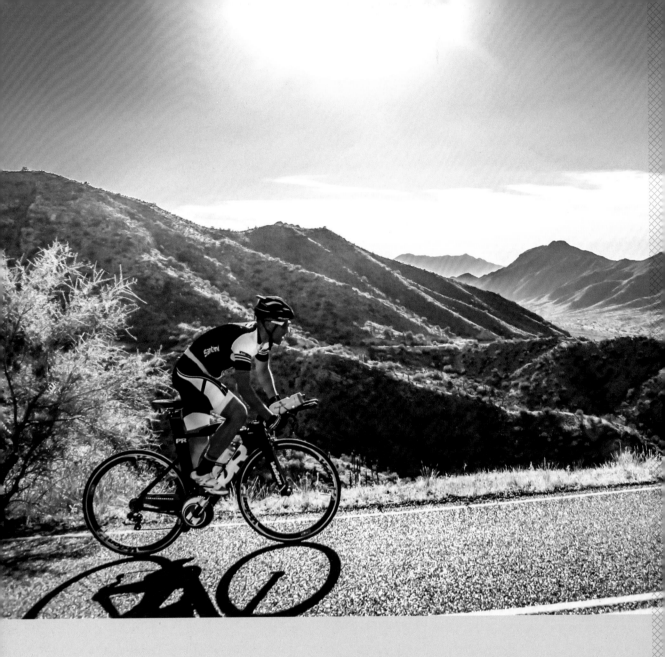

base! As you start ramping up your workouts, your body will reach into itself, tapping in to stores of vitamins and minerals for the ability to push through and recover. You'll do well to stock your body with nutrients in advance—in fact, you should focus all of your attention on eating nutrient-dense foods as an ongoing lifestyle.

The nutrient-dense foods that I have the athletes I work with reach for day after day—and that the recipes in the back of the book are based on—are fish, lean meats, lean dairy, fruits, vegetables, nuts, seeds, and legumes.

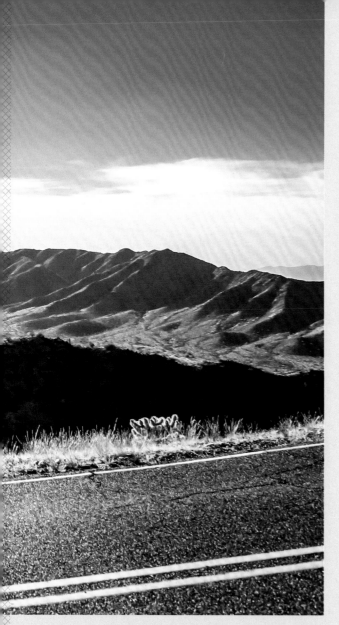

(see page 25). Furthermore, with some minor modifications discussed herein, a diet based on these foods is sustainable. It isn't so limited that it's hard to live life; you'll likely be able to find something on any restaurant menu that fits the bill. We don't always have total control over our dietary options, but these guidelines are helpful for making smart choices wherever you are.

Other less-nutrient-dense foods like breads, pasta, and sports bars serve an important role for the athlete but should be consumed at specific times in order to reap the potential benefits; otherwise they're just empty calories. In general, you should steer clear of any processed foods and anything enhanced with refined sugars, pumped full of animal and vegetable fats, or loaded with secondary salts. The goal is to consume foods in whole forms, as close to the source as possible, in order to get their full load of nutrients into your body, unless there is a specific purpose not to do so. In short, it comes down to the plain and simple fact that extraordinary athletic feats require extraordinary fuels. We will discuss this concept further later, but my use of the word *extraordinary* as it applies to food refers to grains and refined-sugar fuels not found in nature. These extraordinary fuels that I recommend have ideal macronutrient profiles to optimize athletic performance, although they don't necessarily promote a healthy lifestyle on their own without exercise. For example, eating a sports nutrition bar just before a difficult training session is very different from eating the same bar just before going to bed. It is my aim to help you understand why, so you'll be able to make good choices on your own.

Throughout the book, I'll refer to these as our *core foods*, since they're the foundation of all we eat. These foods provide us with a complete macronutrient (proteins, carbohydrates, and fats) profile, and also set the basis for meeting our micronutrient (vitamins and minerals) needs

OPTIMIZATION PHASES

An athlete's physical potential is not just a function of inborn talent and physical and mental preparation. It also depends on eating habits throughout each stage of fitness development and over the long haul. Understanding this concept and using it well can give you a significant leg up on the competition—whether you're competing against other individual athletes, teams, or simply the clock.

Working on the base of healthy eating that you've already established, you'll need to add to that diet once your training phase begins by targeting pre-, during-, and postworkout meals and/or snacks that will support performance. This is when some of the normally "extraordinary" foods may be incorporated. There is definitely a time and a place when and where a sports drink, though clearly very processed and chock-full of sugars, is exactly what the body needs. These engineered beverages do a great job supporting the body in workouts and races when used in thoughtful ways. And the same is true of other processed products, like energy bars (for a longer discussion, see page 57).

THE CORE FOODS

Again, our core foods are fish, lean meats, lean dairy, fruits, vegetables, nuts, seeds, and legumes.

Fish: Fatty or lean, fish is an excellent source of protein. Fatty cold-water fish like salmon is high in omega-3 fatty acids, a very important nutrient for athletes (see more on page 32).

Lean meats: Leans meats are animal proteins that are low in saturated fats. Chicken breast, pork tenderloin, lean cuts of beef—these sorts of foods are great to eat. Foods like bacon, pork belly, chicken thighs, and brisket should be eaten sparingly.

Lean dairy: Any dairy product that's low in saturated fat is great to consume. Look for low-fat yogurt, cheeses (feta, goat cheese, and cottage cheese, for example), and milk. Be careful with low-fat fruit-flavored yogurts, though, as they tend to be very high in added sugar (see Core Ratio on page 20, which discusses how to deal with this).

Fruits: Excellent sources of vitamins and minerals, fruits also provide natural carbohydrates and are high in antioxidants. Different fruits have different mixes of nutrients, so try to eat a wide variety. Some tasty and beneficial ones are blueberries, raspberries, prunes, strawberries, bananas, pineapple, mangoes, and dried figs.

Vegetables: Just like fruits, vegetables are nutrient powerhouses, as they are chock-full of vitamins, minerals, antioxidants, and natural carbs. Again, aim to eat many different types of veggies; some of my top picks are broccoli, red bell peppers, asparagus, spinach, sweet potatoes, butternut squash, and purple and green cabbage.

Nuts: An excellent source of minerals, nuts also provide healthy fats, often including the much-needed omega-3 fatty acids. Most athletes opt

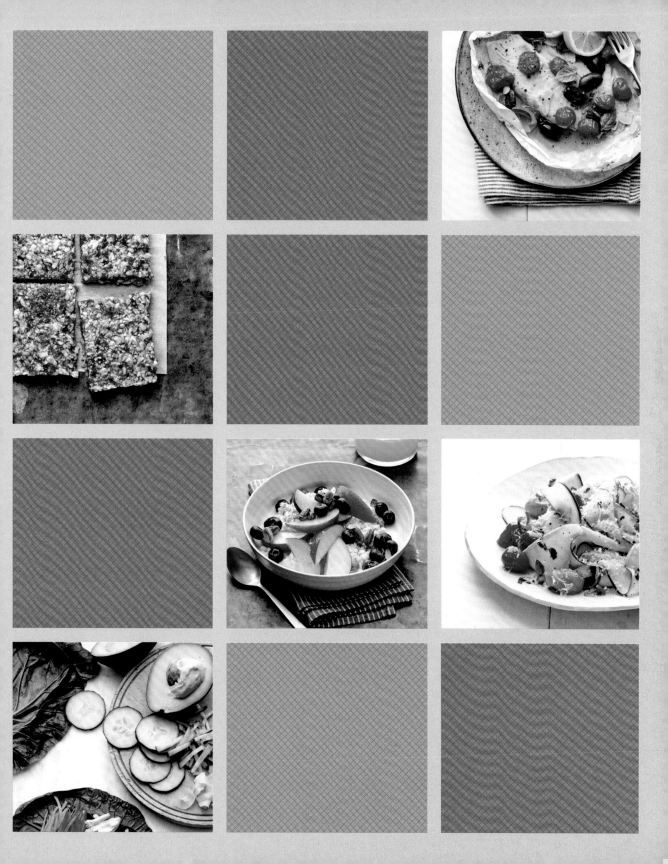

for almonds, and these are fine, but I prefer to choose nuts that contain omega-3 fatty acids (which almonds do not). Walnuts, for example, are high in omega-3s; also, check out the Fruit and Nut Energy Blend on page 155. Brazil nuts and macadamias are also good choices.

Seeds: Packed with minerals such as magnesium, iron, potassium, and selenium, seeds are an important source of nourishment. Seeds should be eaten raw, since their nutritional components break down pretty quickly once they're exposed to heat. They can, however, be soaked, ground, or mashed and still maintain their original nutritional nature. Great options in this category include chia, pumpkin, flax, sesame, and sunflower seeds.

Legumes: Peas, beans, lentils, and peanuts are members of the legume family. Legumes provide excellent protein, dietary fiber, carbohydrates, and micronutrients such as folate, thiamin, manganese, magnesium, potassium, and iron. Legumes also contain starches, which help the body convert food to energy more efficiently and effectively.

CORE RATIO

With the hectic lives we lead, we can't possibly eat core foods 100% of the time. I often find myself in a place where I don't have my own snacks and I'm hungry! So sometimes we have to rely on packaged foods. And some of them can help us reach our goal of stabilizing blood sugar levels and provide good macro- and micronutrients to promote recovery, while satiating our tummies. I've developed what I call the core ratio to help recognize which packaged foods are better than others to eat when in a pinch. See the equation.

This simple equation attempts to magnify the blood sugar impact of a food's carbohydrates by double-counting the sugars. It then also leverages the low blood sugar response of fiber by subtracting it from the carbohydrate count. This numerator is then divided by the combined fat and protein, as both of these have a diluting effect on blood sugar response (since they digest more slowly). Foods that have a core ratio of less than 2 pass the test as long as they have mostly natural or organic ingredients. One other thing to look out for is saturated fat; aim for less than 5 grams per serving in packaged foods.

By using the core ratio, you'll find several types of chips, breads, wraps, burritos, and even a pizza or two that are decent choices. For meals and snacks, make sure that each item meets the core ratio versus just looking at the combined total. In other words, if I want to eat cheese and crackers, I'll check that both the cheese and the crackers are in accordance with the core ratio requirements, are under 5 grams of saturated fat, and contain natural ingredients.

$$\text{CORE RATIO} = (\text{SUGAR} + \text{TOTAL CARBOHYDRATES} - \text{FIBER}) / (\text{TOTAL FAT} + \text{PROTEIN})$$

TOTAL FAT
The amount of fat included in each serving (in grams).

SATURATED FAT
Look for foods that have less than 5 grams of saturated fat.

SUGAR
Aim to eat foods that don't have a lot of added sugars. Natural sugars are okay.

Nutrition Facts

Serving Size 8 crackers (28g)
(1 serving = 2 full cracker sheets)
Servings Per Container About 16

Amount Per Serving

Calories 120   **Calories from Fat** 20
                                     % Daily Value*

Total Fat 2.5g	4%
Saturated Fat 0g	0%
Polyunsaturated Fat 0g	
Monounsaturated Fat 1g	
Cholesterol 0mg	0%
Sodium 140mg	6%
Total Carbohydrate 22g	7%
Dietary Fiber 1g	4%
Sugars 7g	
Protein 2g	
Vitamin A 0%	Vitamin C 0%
Calcium 2%	Iron 6%

* Percent Daily Values are based on a 2,000 calorie diet. Your daily values may be higher or lower depending on your calorie needs.

	Calories	2,000	2,500
Total Fat	Less than	65g	80g
Sat Fat	Less than	20%	25g
Cholesterol	Less than	300mg	300mg
Sodium	Less than	2,400 mg	2,400mg
Total Carbohydrate		300g	375g
Dietary Fiber		25g	30g

TOTAL CARBOHYDRATE
This figure totals dietary fiber, sugars, and other types of sugar or starch in a food product.

PROTEIN
A protein-rich food contains 7 grams of protein or more per serving.

(S + C − FIBER)   **(F + P)**
7 + 22 − 1 = 28 grams   2.5 + 2 = 4.5 grams

28 / 4.5 = 6.2

***NOT* CORE FRIENDLY**

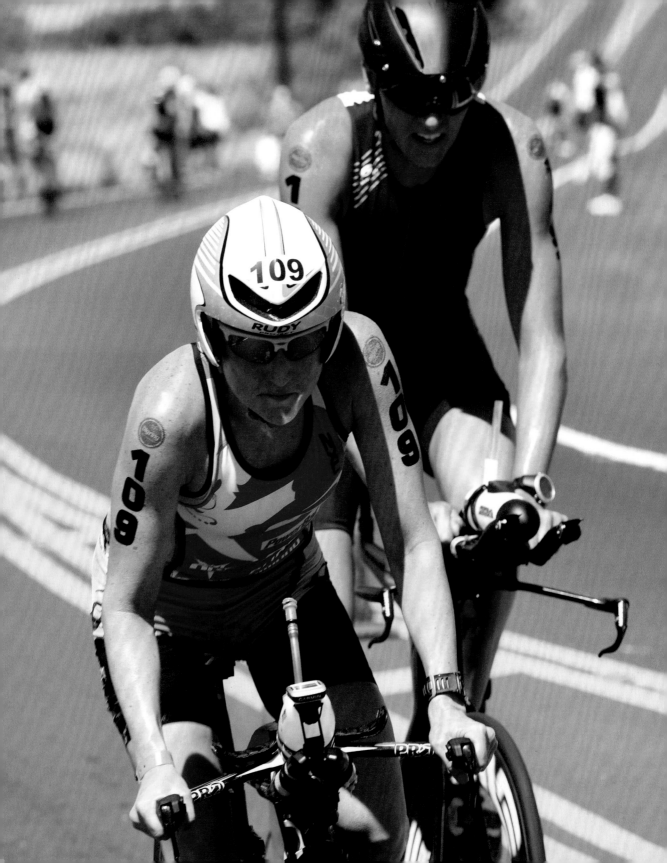

2

ADAPTING
NUTRITION FOR THE
ATHLETE

WHEN YOU BEGIN TRAINING FOR ENDURANCE SPORTS, you'll start burning lots of calories during workouts and eating more food to keep up with your increased activity. But wait! Don't just grab the nearest decent-sounding food and chow down—even if the packaging says it's a "sports" food. Be mindful of what you reach for, since the road to excellent performance is greatly affected by our food choices. All of this puts the athlete into a bit of a catch-22. Athletes require more nutrient density in order to aid in recovery and maintain systemic health, so that their next training session can be as valuable as possible, and so on. The issue is that athletes spend so much time training that they have less and less time to take in these important foods. For this reason, a lunchtime bagel, which contains 80 grams of carbohydrate and few other nutrients, is a missed opportunity, when a nice salad would have been the much better option to get perhaps the same amount of carbohydrate, with much more nutrient density. Every time you eat or drink, you have a chance to give your body something it needs. But first, it's important to understand what those needs are.

MACRONUTRIENTS AND MICRONUTRIENTS

Understanding athletic nutrition begins with learning that macronutrients are proteins, carbohydrates, and fats, and micronutrients are vitamins and minerals. We need a wide variety of macronutrients and micronutrients every day, and we get them through the foods that we eat. I have never been a fan of counting or even reading calories—athletes need to be much smarter than that! I think of the development of nutrition knowledge as occurring in four stages. The first stage uses a points system; points are simple to use for quantifying how much food is consumed, and they don't consider the content of food (or nutrient density and loss of muscle versus fat is not considered). The second stage uses calories; similar to points, counting calories requires little knowledge of or care regarding nutrient density or body composition. These first two stages of understanding are not appropriate for athletes! They are way too simplistic and discount the things that matter most. Stage three is an understanding of macronutrients. Proteins, carbohydrates, and fats each have their own primary functions, and knowing when and why to consume each is important to an athlete's daily objectives, as well as long-term objectives regarding body composition. Finally, the fourth stage gets us to micronutrients, or understanding vitamins and minerals. This is when you know that a 20-gram carbohydrate serving of blueberries has more nutrient density than the same 20-gram carbohydrate serving of melon. With this level of nutrition knowledge, athletes and nonathletes are armed with logic they can implement throughout life.

MACRONUTRIENTS

I'm guessing that most readers already know the basics of what proteins, carbohydrates, and fats are. We need to consume all of these macronutrients via our food daily, and we can manipulate the ratios of each to achieve different goals of body composition (the amounts of muscle, fat, bone, and water in our bodies). Let's take a closer look at each, from the point of view of endurance athletes.

Proteins

Proteins are, quite simply, a linked group of amino acids. They are large molecules and an essential part of the structural components of all living organisms—things like hair, collagen, and muscle. We consume protein from two primary sources: plants and animals. Unlike fat and carbohydrate, protein is not stored in the body in large quantities. The protein that we eat is used as we eat it. For this reason, as well as many others, athletes need to eat good, clean, and efficient sources of protein, meaning those that are readily absorbed by the body and that closely match the amino acid profile of human muscle tissue.

The proteins that are best absorbed by the body include those found in whey, whole soybeans, soybean milk, cow's milk, chicken eggs, and buckwheat. Each of these absorbs at a rate of about 90% of its potential. As athletes, we want food sources that our bodies can access easily, like a team of workers reconstructing a damaged building. Our protein sources are our workers, ready with hammers and nails to repair any damage that may have occurred during the storm of our respective workouts. The protein

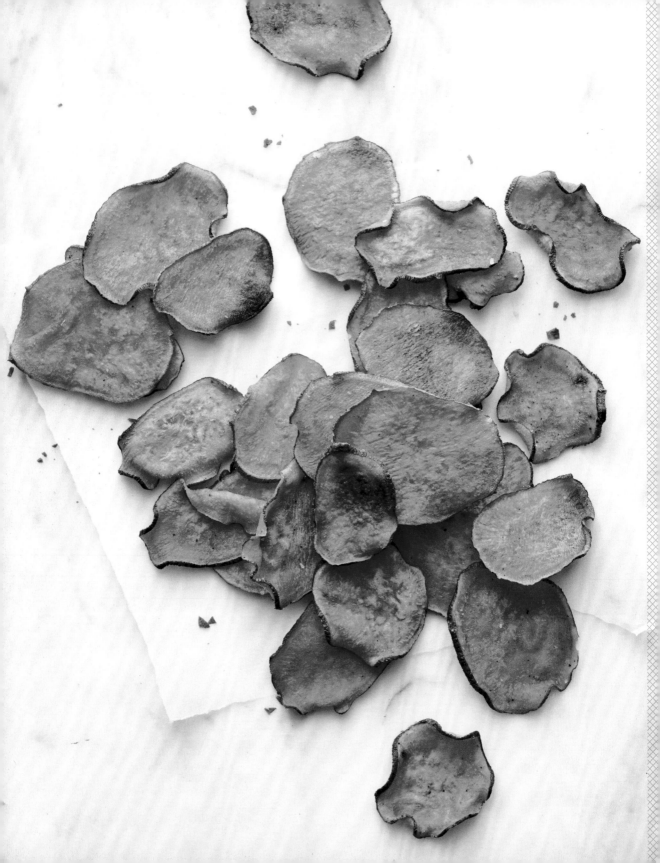

sources mentioned here are probably the most efficient that the body can absorb, and they contain the raw building blocks the human body needs to repair muscle tissue. Athletes often rely on whey and egg proteins the most, because proteins that come from animal sources are the most complete. Plant-based proteins can also repair damage but will probably have to borrow other amino acids in the body to do so. Having said that, vegans and vegetarians can also excel at endurance sports; it just takes some extra hard work and focus to get the amino acids they require. I like to have vegans and vegetarians supplement with L-leucene, which is difficult to obtain in proper quantities without having animal sources of protein.

Carbohydrates

Carbohydrates play the largest daily role in meeting the body's energy demands. They help restore glycogen, the body's most raw and readily available fuel source, which is stored in both the liver and muscle. Carbohydrates come in many forms, and the term makes most people immediately think of such foods as bread, pasta, and candy. Our culture has made this macronutrient almost synonymous with the term *grain*, but foods like sweet potatoes, bananas, and melons also contain carbs. Grains—especially highly processed foods made from grains—are generally not very nutrient dense and create large blood sugar swings. Fruits and vegetables, on the other hand, are packed with nutrients and are truly the best sources for valuable carbohydrates. If you take away nothing else from this discussion, realize that you can get plenty of

carbs from fruits and vegetables. *Carbohydrate does not mean grain!*

Fats

Fats, like the other macronutrients, come in many forms, and as with proteins and carbs, your focus should be on seeking out the fats that will give you the best bang for your nutrition buck. Contrary to popular belief, your body doesn't know the difference between 40 grams of fat from a half stick of butter or 40 grams of fat from a salmon steak. These two foods will affect your body composition the same way; however, the fat in the salmon steak will reduce inflammation, cushion your joints, and act as an antioxidant. The fat from the butter will do none of that, rather it will clog your arteries. Beneficial fats include omega-3 fatty acids and monounsaturated fats such as omega-9. Polyunsaturated fats such as omega-6 are also beneficial, but most of us get plenty of those from the foods we eat already (see page 32 for a full discussion on omega-3s and other fatty acids).

MICRONUTRIENTS

Micronutrients are like magic. Maybe that's a little over the top, but these vitamins and minerals can be significantly beneficial to the body, especially when consumed in a smart way. All of our core foods contain lots of micronutrients, and in mixing and varying the diet, we can make great progress toward consuming all of the essential ones.

Electrolytes

Electrolytes are minerals that hold an electric charge. They are important to athletes because

CAFFEINE
COFFEE VS. GREEN TEA

Caffeine is the drug of choice for most people these days to cope with our overstressed and under-rested lives. Because higher-content caffeine sources like coffee increase systematic stress, I like to treat coffee as a grain or a refined sugar. That is, just as grains and refined sugars raise blood sugar quickly, caffeine has a swift and intense impact on the nervous system. This impact is felt by the adrenal system and is a stress just like other stresses in a person's life. With that, I recommend avoiding coffee for day-to-day consumption between workouts. As an alternative to coffee, green tea—which generally contains much less caffeine and has high levels of one of the most powerful antioxidants (epigallocatechin gallate, also known as EGCG)—is perfect for a quick pick-me-up. Try to keep caffeine intake from all sources below 200 milligrams per day, and 1,000 milligrams per week for men and 800 milligrams per week for women. I have worked with thousands of athletes to remove coffee and other caffeine-rich foods and drinks from their daily habits, and almost every single one of them can't believe how much better they feel once they adjust. However, there is a time and a place for higher-caffeine-content drinks and sports products; see page 40.

they affect your muscle function and the way your body stores water. The five big electrolytes in the body are:

- **SODIUM:** regulates water in your body
- **POTASSIUM:** regulates the heart and the muscles' ability to function
- **MAGNESIUM:** helps the muscles relax
- **CALCIUM:** drives the muscles' ability to contract; also necessary for bone health
- **CHLORIDE:** also helps regulate water in your body

As endurance athletes, we are most concerned with sodium and magnesium, so we'll look a little closer at these two here.

SODIUM: Of the five big electrolytes, sodium is by far the biggest driver for endurance athletes and is the most common limiter of possible performance on race day. I think of sodium as a short-term electrolyte because you can deplete and replete it rapidly. I think of potassium and magnesium as longer-term electrolytes because they take time to build up and deplete within the body. So with sodium we must constantly think of what's being expended so that we are adequately resupplying our body with it.

When we train and race, our bodies push fluids to the surface of the skin to encourage evaporation, which cools us down. The lost fluid (our sweat) contains electrolytes—in particular, large amounts of sodium. We also lose significant amounts of sodium via urination. The losses of this electrolyte incurred through sweat and urine are substantial, and most athletes underestimate these losses. I recommend that athletes tally their planned hourly race-day sodium intake and measure it against the realization that most athletes lose between 500 and 4,000 milligrams of sodium per hour during endurance sport races. To get a reasonable estimate of your specific needs, assume a loss of 450 to 700 milligrams of sodium per 16 ounces of sweat lost (I've found this to be pretty average). If you have experienced muscle cramping during your racing in the past, err to the higher side of this range. Using this sodium concentration and estimated fluid loss based on the urination rule of thumb (see page 78), you can get a pretty good idea of your actual sodium needs. During a race, most athletes require 500 to 600 milligrams of sodium per 24 ounces of sports drink, plus the sodium in any additional products, such as gels, bars, and sodium tablets. This brings the minimum requirement to about 500 milligrams, and the maximum as high as 4,000 milligrams. An athlete's sodium requirement is primarily determined by the sweat rate (see page 78) and can vary by as much as a factor of four between a low-sweat-rate person and a high-sweat-rate person.

The simplest thing most athletes can do is to choose a sports drink that provides an ample amount of sodium such that—as long as sweat rates are matched with commensurate fluid intake—sodium needs will be met in 95% of cases. This makes for an easy-to-follow fueling plan. And yet, the most significant race-day issue that athletes encounter with respect to sodium is in using drinks that do not contain enough sodium and/or not drinking enough fluids. Many athletes simply do not realize how much they sweat and end up short in both sodium and fluids. Regardless of the athlete's sodium needs, it is not a bad policy to *always* carry extra sodium on race day (see page 37 for more on supplements).

Lastly, for hot-weather race days, consider including an acute sodium load during the final 24 hours before race day during the carbohydrate load. The additional sodium will allow your body to retain extra fluids and sodium, which come in handy on race day. To properly execute a sodium load of this nature, simply focus on sodium-rich carbohydrate sources during the carbohydrate load period. Items like pretzels and sports drinks are perfect! For most athletes, 3,000 milligrams of sodium the day before a race, gleaned from the foods you eat, is enough.

On pages 30–31 is a table I regularly use with my athletes to calculate sodium losses, and therefore also their needs.

MAGNESIUM: It took me almost 15 years to understand the impact that magnesium could have for endurance sports. It's an interesting electrolyte. Athletes who have experienced foot or calf cramps when they sleep, or even foot cramping during early-morning swims, are likely deficient in magnesium. I once had an athlete who often began cramping at the starting line— before his races had even started. I scratched my head for years trying to figure out why, and eventually I realized that given his high sweat rate and focus on staying hydrated as we got close to races, he had flushed magnesium and potentially other electrolytes from his body. If you have had similar experiences, simply add to your diet a daily serving of pumpkin seeds, the richest natural source of magnesium. In addition to eating pumpkin seeds, those with chronic

SAMPLE FLUID & SODIUM ANALYSES FOR BIKING

SPORT	WEIGHT BEFORE TRAINING	WEIGHT AFTER TRAINING	WEIGHT CHANGE *1lb = 16oz*	TOTAL FLUID CONSUMED
1 Bike Indoors	150 lb.	149.2 lb.	0.8 lb.	22 oz.
2 Race Conditions (80°F, sunny)	150.26 lb.	149.2 lb.	1.1 lb.	22 oz.
3 Average Person/ Average Conditions	150 lb.	149.3 lb.	0.7 lb.	20 oz.

RECOMMENDED FLUID & SODIUM INTAKES

	OLYMPIC (2.5 hours)		HALF IRON (5 hours)	
	FLUID PER HOUR	SODIUM PER HOUR	FLUID PER HOUR	SODIUM PER HOUR
1 Bike Indoors	21 oz.	400 mg.	25 oz.	500 mg.
2 Race Conditions (80°F, sunny)	25 oz.	500 mg.	29 oz.	600 mg.
3 Average Person/ Average Conditions	17 oz.	300 mg.	21 oz.	400 mg.

SWEAT LOSS	EXERCISE TIME (min.)	SWEAT LOSS PER HOUR	ASSUMED SODIUM per 16 oz of sweat	SODIUM LOSS (mg) per hour	MAXIMUM ACCEPTABLE LIQUID DEFICIT (body weight x 2%) x 16
34.8 oz.	60	34.8 oz.	500 mg	1088 mg.	48 oz.
39 oz.	60	39 oz.	500 mg.	1218 mg.	48 oz.
31.2 oz.	60	31.2 oz.	500 mg.	975 mg.	48 oz.

IRON
(11 hours)

FLUID PER HOUR	SODIUM PER HOUR
30 oz.	600 mg.
34 oz.	700 mg.
26 oz.	500 mg.

ALCOHOL

I am often asked where alcohol fits in to the core diet, and especially as it applies to athletes. I keep a reasonable approach to alcohol that takes into account that most people are going to want to have a drink now and then. I also realize that the abuse of alcohol can have very real, negative consequences on an athlete's performance. Over the years, I have developed the following sensible approach, which also dovetails well with the nutrition periodization concepts discussed on page 64. Here's what I follow and recommend:

• **OFF SEASON:** No more than 2 drinks per day.

• **DURING TRAINING:** No more than 2 drinks, 2 days per week.

• **FINAL 6 WEEKS BEFORE A MAJOR RACE:** No alcohol at all.

Note that by "drink," I mean red wine or light beer. I recommend that athletes stay away from hard alcohol entirely, because it's a slippery slope! Hard alcohol gets you tipsy faster, which makes it easier to make poor food consumption decisions and/or drink too much. It's also a lot easier to get dehydrated, since liquor contains less fluid per gram of alcohol.

cramping issues can try soaking for 15 minutes in an Epsom salts bath, using 2 cups of Epsom salts per bath and water at a temperature of 95 to 100°F. Epsom salts are rich in magnesium, which is readily absorbed through the skin, and they help relax your muscles, too.

Omega-3s

Omega-3s are polyunsaturated fatty acids that are very important for the endurance athlete. Omega-3s are essential fatty acids—"essential" because the body requires them for good health but is unable to create them on its own or by synthesizing other compounds. Therefore—you guessed it—we have to ingest them.

Omega-3s have a close relation, one that very few people are familiar with: omega-6 fatty acids. Also essential fatty acids, omega-6s are necessary for the body to function properly, but the body cannot create them on its own. So, again, we have to ingest them. But why don't we ever see them at the pharmacy? Unlike omega-3s, omega-6s aren't available as a supplement. Why is that?

Well, it turns out that the modern American diet is chock-full of omega-6 fatty acids, since our processed foods use so much vegetable oil. Omega-6s are also found in poultry, eggs, avocados, nuts, cereals, and whole-grain breads, as well as many other foods. But because of the ubiquitous vegetable oils, we have more than enough omega-6 in our bodies.

Research has shown that the human body

functions best with a balanced ratio of omega-6s to omega-3s in the range of 3 to 1 or 4 to 1. Today's American diet, infused with vegetable oils from every angle, is virtually entirely void of omega-3s, and has therefore created a situation where we are ingesting omega-6 fatty acids at an alarming rate of 20 to 1, and often as much as 30 to 1. A 20-to-1 ratio means that for every twenty instances of ingestible inflammation, we provide our bodies with only one counterbalancing instance. Put another way, more than 95% of the essential fatty acids consumed are promoting inflammation!

Remember having a piggy bank as a kid? Your little brother or sister probably had one, too. Chances are that you had a grandparent who would come over and rattle some change out of his pocket or her purse. It was such a fun time in life! But there was always that unfortunate condition of having to split the change with your sibling. Annoying, yes, but the cost of doing business as a 6-year-old. So Grandpa would pull four shiny quarters from his pocket, and hand two to you and two to your brother or sister, and you would run off to deposit them into the pig for the joy of hearing the sound of the coins hitting the bottom, or better yet, hitting other already-deposited coins. A natural evolution of fairness and balance, right? Every one was happy! Well, imagine if Grandpa didn't fish out four quarters. Instead it was a mix of quarters, dimes, nickels, and pennies. Maybe not as exciting as shiny new quarters, but money is money. Our modern-day omega-6 to omega-3 intake is the equivalent of Grandpa handing your annoying little brother three quarters, three dimes, two nickels, and five pennies, and giving you a nickel and a penny. What

THE MANY BENEFITS OF
OMEGA-3S

Omega-3 fatty acids have been shown not only to reduce the inflammatory effects of omega-6s, stress, and pollutants on our organs, but also to reduce the inflammation associated with arthritis and other joint-related pain conditions. They help cushion the joints. A 2007 study published in the *Journal of the American College of Nutrition* found that 300 milligrams of krill oil (an excellent source of omega-3s) each day greatly reduced joint inflammation, joint pain, joint stiffness, and functional joint impairment after only 7 days of use. The benefits were even better defined after 14 days of use. This was true for both people with rheumatoid arthritis and those with osteoarthritis. Above and beyond the anti-inflammatory nature of omega-3 fatty acids, this micronutrient has other wide-ranging benefits when consumed, including a decreased risk of coronary heart disease and lowered cholesterol levels. Researchers in the cancer, depression, and attention deficit/hyperactivity disorder (ADHD) fields, just to name a few, have seen promising results from their studies of the effects of omega-3s in these areas as well. So what are you waiting for? Start upping your intake today!

would happen? You would throw your six cents to the ground and run from the room crying. Why? Because Grandpa wasn't being fair. He created an imbalance between you and your little brother.

Our contemporary diet is like that unfair grandparent who creates turmoil in the house. The extreme imbalance of omega-6 fatty acids to omega-3s is causing problems within our bodies. Group this dietary inflammation-promoting imbalance with increased family, work, and general life stresses (all of which are inflammation-promoting), and then add it to a world that has seen pollution levels increase (another inflammation promoter) at

levels beyond mention, and we have quite a predicament. In this equation, the one thing that we have the most control over—our diets—is, from an inflammatory standpoint, doing us more harm than good.

We can really help our bodies be healthier and perform their functions best by aiming to even out the ratio of omega-6s to omega-3s via the foods that we put into our bodies. This ratio promotes an atmosphere where the body exists in a healthy and typically less inflamed state. In general, it promotes an anti-inflammatory response throughout the body, which helps maintain a healthy circulatory system. This means that oxygen, carbon dioxide, red blood cells, white blood cells, serum, water, sugars, toxins, and the like are constantly moving. The circulatory system is the body's river. When it moves at a nice steady rate, everything remains clean and healthy. Like a river, when circulation is slowed, then pollutants such as carbon dioxide and toxins are allowed to build up. This creates an adverse atmosphere for general health— acutely so for athletes who are trying to recover from day-to-day workouts and training. A healthy ratio of omega-6 to omega-3 fatty acids keeps the river flowing smoothly, constantly flushing harmful toxins.

So how do we go about reducing this omega-6 to omega-3 ratio by more than four times? This seems like a tough task, but it's not as complicated as it looks. I recommend a very simple two-pronged approach to shift the ratio from 20 to 1 to 4 to 1. Reduce the numerator (omega-6s in your diet), and increase the denominator (omega-3s in your diet).

A CLOSER LOOK AT

OILS

All oils are not created equally when it comes to omegas. Both olive and coconut oils are far superior options to even canola oil. One tablespoon of olive oil contains about an eighth of the omega-6s of canola oil, a twentieth of those of soybean oil, and a twenty-fifth of those of corn oil. Choosing olive oil over these other oils would make a tremendous difference to the omega ratio in your body. But even better is coconut oil, which has about four times less omega-6 fatty acids than olive oil! Just be careful with the amount of saturated fat in coconut oil.

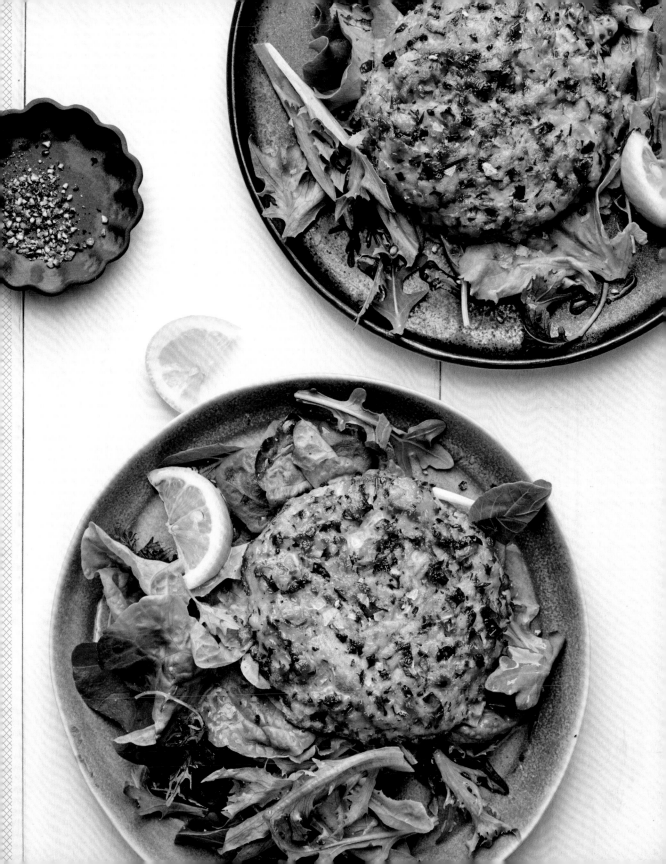

1. **Lose the processed foods!** Processed foods are loaded with vegetable oils, such as soybean, corn, canola, and cottonseed. Of these, canola oil is the least egregious, with a tablespoon containing about a third of pro-inflammatory omega-6 fatty acids as compared with a tablespoon of corn oil, and about half that of soybean oil.
2. **Focus on the core foods:** fish, lean meats, lean dairy, fruits, vegetables, nuts, seeds, and legumes. Because the core foods are not processed with added oils, they are by default lower in omega-6s. In addition, several of the core foods—such as salmon, avocado, and walnuts—contain lots of omega-3s.

1. **Add flaxseeds and flax oil to your foods.** Flax is a tremendous source of omega-3 fatty acids and many other nutrients, too. A 100-gram (3½-ounce) serving of flax contains more than 18 grams of protein, 143% of the

DIFFERENT TYPES OF
OMEGA-3S

There are three different types of omega-3 fatty acids: EPA (eicosapentaenoic), DHA (docosahexaenoic), and ALA (a-Linolenic). They are responsible for fortifying the systems that run the show in our bodies. DHA is a primary structural component of the human brain, cerebral cortex, skin, sperm, testicles, and retina. That's pretty important stuff! EPA and DHA come from marine oils, whereas ALA is found in plant oils. It turns out that we don't have too much trouble getting the necessary ALA intake, but EPA and DHA sources are much more limited. In essence, we don't eat enough fish! Cultures that center life, and therefore diets, on the fishing industry are much more likely to get the necessary levels of EPA and DHA. We have all seen those rare stories on CNN or *60 Minutes* that study people in the hinterlands of some underdeveloped country who live well past the age of 100 because they eat nothing but homegrown vegetables and freshly caught fish. I'm not saying that we should quit our jobs, move to a far-off land, and buy a heavy-duty fishing net. But we should eat more fish. Keep in mind that although the plant-based omega-3 options are good, your body has to go through some work to convert these fatty acids to the anti-inflammatory agents EPA and DHA. Flax, walnuts, and avocados are all great sources of ALA, but they won't be as effective in raising EPA and DHA levels as the animal-based sources such as salmon.

Recommended Dietary Allowance (RDA) of thiamin, 13% of riboflavin, 21% of niacin, 20% of pantothenic acid, and 36% of good old-fashioned vitamin B_6. And that's just the vitamins. It gets even more impressive when we take a look at the mineral profile: 26% of the RDA for calcium, 44% of iron, 17% of potassium, 46% of zinc, 92% of phosphorus, and a whopping 110% of the RDA for magnesium. So flax is beneficial to consume overall, but it will also greatly contribute to correcting the ratio of omega-6s to omega-3s; that same 100-gram serving contains 42 grams of fat, mostly from omega-3 fatty acids. And flax's own omega-6 to omega-3 ratio is very impressive: 4 to 1! So there are significantly more omega-3 fatty acids in flaxseed than there are omega-6s.

2. **Choose cold-water fish.** Fish that live in cold water—such as salmon, anchovies, and rainbow trout, to name a few popular and widely available options—are high in omega-3s. A 6-ounce portion of rainbow trout can contain as much as 2 grams of omega-3 fatty acids. Wild salmon is even better, with 3.2 grams, which is an entire daily serving's worth! Cringe now, but sardines are even more potent, with 3.4 grams per 6-ounce serving. Some other, maybe less-known and less-available, options are Pacific mackerel, sable, whitefish, bluefin tuna, and Atlantic herring. Try to consume cold-water fish twice a week to help increase your omega-3 intake.

3. **Stock up on walnuts.** Just ¼ cup—the equivalent of about a handful—of walnuts contains about 2.7 grams of omega-3 fatty acids. And while

there are certainly omega-6 fatty acids in ¼ cup of nuts, the omega-6 to omega-3 ratio is great, at 4.2 to 1. Chia seeds and flaxseeds have even lower ratios but are not as practical to eat regularly. For instance, chia seeds and flaxseeds have remarkably low omega ratios: 0.3 to 1 and 0.2 to 1, respectively. The popular almond? Almost no omega-3s at all!

4. **Take a fish oil supplement.** I know how hard it is to increase omega-3 levels by diet alone, so I always have my athletes incorporate a fish oil supplement as well. See page 38 for more on supplements.

SUPPLEMENTS

It's pretty amazing to me that we can—and many people do—get most of what our bodies need to be healthy functioning machines in pill form. Low on iron? Don't eat a steak! Take this little black triangular pill of ferrous sulfate. Low on vitamin D because you're not getting enough sun? Don't bother going outside; there is a small football-shaped orb for that. Vitamin C? No need to eat a small orange, which has about 50 milligrams of vitamin C, or a little more than half of the recommended daily intake. Just plop a packet of Emergen-C into water, and you can have 1,000 milligrams, about 1,667% of the recommended daily intake. I don't think that supplements are totally bogus, but I think we can be smarter about getting essential nutrients than merely taking them in engineered forms. Besides, these products have terrible absorption rates compared with what's found in food.

And yet, while I'm a huge advocate of eating good, whole foods—and a wide variety of them—to get all the nutrients you need, there are times when supplements can help. There are a few that I recommend to my athletes, but it's a small number, and mostly items I would consider more akin to "concentrated" food than something engineered. Keep in mind that the FDA does not regulate supplements. Make sure that you purchase them from reliable sources, since some products on the market have been proven to be fake (in other words, you don't get what you pay for). And many companies try to promote their wares based on claims that a product can enhance a body in a particular manner. I call that "the supplement fallacy." All the supplement will do is take a body from being deficient in a certain nutrient, and therefore sometimes unable to function as it should, to a nondeficient state. The company's superhuman promises fall totally flat.

For years, I was really into supplements—I even worked in a shop that was dedicated to them! And so, after spending lots of money experimenting with a wide array of powders and pills, I can honestly say that most of them have no performance-enhancing quality at all. In the following paragraphs I outline the handful of supplements I do recommend.

Whey Protein

Whey protein powder is a basic supplement and food item. Whey protein contains a quality profile of amino acids that closely matches the amino acid content found in human muscle tissue. This supplement is most useful to help enhance dietary protein for athletes looking to put on muscle mass, support weight training, and remove strength as a limiter. When choosing a whey protein, look for one with as few artificial ingredients as possible. One such product is by Klean Athlete, and it contains almost 100% whey protein with very limited added ingredients, such as artificial sweeteners and thickening agents.

Dose: *As needed to supplement dietary protein intake for athletes looking to gain muscle. As a rule of thumb, no more than half of an athlete's protein intake should come from nondietary sources. Using whey protein is most convenient in the morning and in the evening before bed. Take no more than 17 to 27 grams in one serving. The research on muscle protein synthesis is pretty strong in showing diminishing benefits after about 27 grams per serving.*

Fish Oil

As discussed on page 32, I like athletes to focus significantly on omega-3 fatty acid intake. I've done years of running blood tests on my athletes to see how much fatty acid consumption they manage, and I don't think I've ever seen someone who hasn't required some dose of a supplement to get their blood levels where we'd like to see them. Most people just don't eat enough foods rich in omega-3! Therefore, for my athletes who may eat fish once or twice a week and maybe walnuts here and there, I have them take a supplement of EPA/DHA daily in the form of fish oil. Having said that, I'm a big believer in supplements being just that, supplements. By that I mean that if you eat salmon on a particular day, there is no need to take a fish oil supplement, too. Only take the supplement on days when you don't get it through dietary sources. But many athletes lose track of this point and just take their supplement every day. That's okay, but I try to encourage them to think more deeply about what they're consuming!

Dose: *Doses of fish oil as a supplement can be specific to the athlete based on training load and normal dietary intake. If you want to really get dialed in, get your blood tested to learn your own fatty acid content. I like for my athletes to have a 4-to-1 or 6-to-1 ratio of eicosapentaenoic acid (EPA) to docosahexaenoic acid (DHA). After working with athletes regularly for many years, I've found that most need a minimum of 2.4 grams of EPA/DHA via fish oil supplementation to be in the ballpark. As mentioned before, don't take the supplement on days when you eat omega-3-rich foods such as salmon.*

Beets (Nitrates)

Beets are known for their high concentrations of nitrate and nitrite, compounds that have performance-enhancing properties, and therefore beet juice is a favorite "supplement" in the racing community. Many vegetables have the same compounds, but not as much as beets. Research over the past several years has shown that increased nitrate and nitrite intake has helped the performance of endurance athletes by improving economy, or the amount of oxygen the body uses for a given workload. Such results are typically seen only through training, so this is amazing stuff!

But before you start slugging beet juice around the clock, you should know that research also shows that there are responders and nonresponders to nitrates and nitrites. If you are a responder, the benefits are big with regard to endurance sport performance. If you are not a responder, a little nutrient-dense beet juice certainly won't hurt you, but you won't see big rewards. Most studies show that only about one or two in twenty athletes are responders, and that the more advanced athletes are less likely to be responders. (Perhaps this phenomenon is due to the fact that the more advanced athletes have already gotten the performance-enhancing adaptations that beet juice targets?)

Dose: *Feel free to drink 8 to 16 ounces of beet juice daily! For specific loading prior to key races, start drinking 10 to 16 ounces of beet juice 5 days before the race (that's the juice of four to five fresh beets). There are also several prepared products on the market, such as Beet Performer, which is 8 ounces of beet juice in a can (it is pasteurized, but research has shown that this process doesn't affect the nitrates and nitrites). There are also a few powdered supplements available; just make sure you know the nitrate and nitrite content of these before trying them. I feel that juice is the best option, especially since you get the added benefit of hydration.*

Race day itself is likely the most beneficial time to dose; many athletes don't realize this. Drink 8 to 16 ounces of beet juice about 30 minutes before the start of the race—which is about as close to the race as possible. This is a time when the powdered supplement may be the best bet, especially if your gut is sensitive to the juice itself.

If your event will last longer than 10 hours, consider taking 8 ounces of beet juice again during the race itself. The half-life of nitrates is about 6 hours, and economy loss due to mechanics degradation (athletes get sloppy and form falls apart) is likely greatest during the later stages of your race. Drinking beet juice

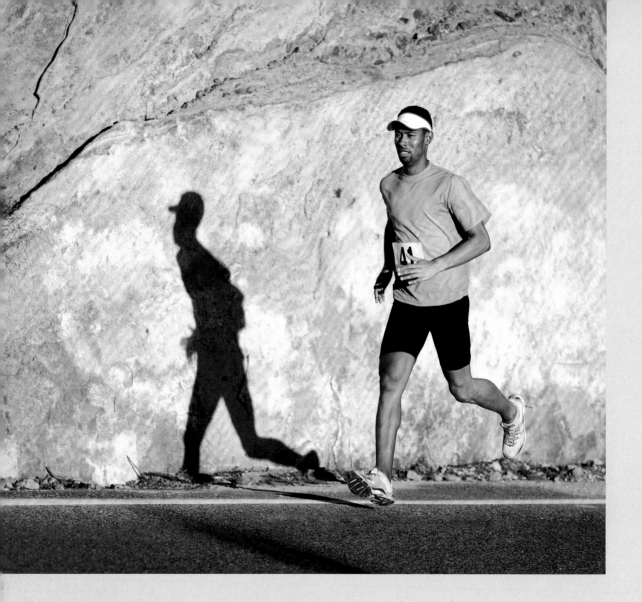

or taking the powder will potentially help combat this degradation by improving economy at the point when your last dose is wearing off. The timing of this dose should be right around 6 hours.

Another time I typically have athletes take larger amounts of beet juice daily is if there is less than 2 weeks between long-distance races such as an IRONMAN or a marathon. During these periods,

we need all the help we can get to recover, and therefore we should continue taking 8 to 16 ounces of beet juice daily.

Caffeine

Caffeine is one of the few proven performance enhancers for race day and in training. However, to get the most benefit from it, and to avoid some of the negative side effects, avoid coffee during your normal training weeks unless it is within 1 hour of a key workout or during a key workout. Try to keep caffeine intake below 200 milligrams per day, and below 1,000 milligrams per week for men and 800 milligrams per week for women. I have found that this balance is practical enough for real life, allowing for noticeable benefits during key sessions without the negative side effects, and helps keep the body sensitive to caffeine so that you'll feel a boost on race day.

During the final 72 hours before race day, it is best to reduce caffeine consumption to zero, in order to realize the full benefits from a race-day performance-enhancing standpoint. If you have more regular caffeine habits, try stepping down your caffeine intake by about 50 milligrams per day until you get to zero 72 hours before the race. This step-down approach is a great way to avoid the negative effects of caffeine withdrawal. During the race itself, gradually increase your caffeine intake as the race progresses. I recommend building caffeine throughout the day to one to two times your body weight in pounds for total caffeine content, in milligrams, for the day (for example, this would be 160 to 320 milligrams for a 160-pound athlete). Since the half-life of caffeine (time it takes for the body to eliminate half of the caffeine) is about 6 hours, for races longer than 6 hours, do not take any caffeine before the race at all. The goal should be to have the blood content of caffeine at its highest as you finish a race. This practice helps you fight fatigue as it sets in, while at the same time not encouraging mispacing the event. For most athletes this means no need for caffeine until

30 minutes before races shorter than 6 hours, and caffeine only starting 6 to 8 hours before the end of races longer than 6 hours. For shorter races like a 5K, since the duration is less than the half-life of caffeine, you can begin caffeine intake 45 minutes to 1 hour before the event.

Dose: *I recommend building caffeine throughout race day up to one to two times your body weight in pounds for total caffeine content in milligrams. For daily consumption, stick with green tea between workout sessions, and save coffee and caffeinated products for just before and during key workouts. Regardless, on a regular basis, keep caffeine intake below 200 milligrams per day, and below 1,000 milligrams per week for men and 800 milligrams per week for women.*

Glutamine

Glutamine (often called L-glutamine) has been around since body builders began using supplements—so for a very long time! It has been studied up and down thousands of times in areas such as athletic performance and GI (gastrointestinal) health. The bottom line is that glutamine is safe, easy to find, and cheap. Research shows that it supports the immune system, protects muscle tissue and aids recovery, and contributes to GI health. Glutamine is a nonessential amino acid, meaning that the body can produce it, and it is also the most abundant amino acid in muscle cells. When you put your body through intense exercise, glutamine stores decrease significantly. If the deficit is too large for the body to replace quickly enough, you will have a deficit for some time. This may mean that you'll experience impaired immunity and a reduced rate of muscle recovery from intense exercise. You can restock this reserve much more quickly by taking glutamine supplements. When training over months and months for endurance races, it's likely you'll find yourself at a deficit at some point, which is why I recommend taking a supplement.

Dose: *Once your weekly training volume reaches about 15 hours, mix 5 grams of glutamine into your postworkout recovery drink each time you take one. If it's a nonworkout day, take 5 grams in the morning and 5 grams in the evening.*

Beta-alanine

A nonessential amino acid like glutamine, beta-alanine has been shown to enhance muscular endurance during cardiovascular exercise, provided that the workout is short in duration and best effort in nature. Its relevance is likely for best-effort exercise durations between 30 seconds and 4 minutes. This amino acid has some research to support its use as a performance enhancer; however, the body of research isn't totally conclusive yet, in my opinion. Given that, I recommend beta-alanine only to athletes who are more aerobic in nature (i.e., they'd rather run a marathon than do quarter-mile repeats on the track) and only when they are training and targeting anaerobic energy systems, such as when they're doing repeats in the 30-second to 4-minute range. If you are not doing this type of training or racing, save your money! This supplement is likely best suited for the road bike racer or cyclocross athlete during race season.

Dose: *Take 4.8 grams of beta-alanine daily, as two separate doses, for 3 weeks. Follow this window*

with doses of 2.4 grams daily, as two separate doses of 1.2 grams each, for up to an additional 9 weeks. Results are typically noticed in 3 to 6 weeks.

Sodium

Even if you have a detailed fueling plan set in stone, it is smart to carry sodium supplements with you during your race as an insurance policy against a deficit. See page 28 for a longer discussion of sodium.

Dose: *Make sure that the sodium supplement you choose contains at least 200 milligrams per capsule. As a rule of thumb, if at any point during a race or training session you feel a muscle twinge or stomach bloating, take a capsule. As an alternative to the customary capsules, BASE Performance makes a freeform version that is applied directly to the tongue. I really like this version, as the absorption starts immediately when it hits your mouth, therefore signaling to the body very quickly that it is coming. The capsule forms bypass that entire natural process.*

Juicing

Once an athlete sticks with a diet based on the core foods with up to 80 or 85% compliance between workout windows, I recommend that he or she begin juicing as a supplement. The point is for the athlete to juice those fruits and veggies he or she doesn't ingest in on a regular basis. Although no athlete should replace whole fruits and veggies with juicing, drinking juices can add great nutrients and antioxidants better than any powder or pill. So if you are confident in your ability to implement the concepts described in this book, try juicing as a bonus to support your training and racing!

BLOOD SUGAR

The aim of this book's approach to food is to maintain a consistent blood sugar level throughout the day. Achieving consistency helps us maintain energy levels and avoid urges to overeat, or binge, out of hunger. And we avoid situations where the body will store unwanted body fat by not giving it more energy than it can burn.

GLYCEMIC LOAD

One way that we try to keep blood sugar levels steady is by minding the glycemic load of the foods we eat. Glycemic load is a calculation that tells us how much of each food will raise our blood sugar. Foods that have low-glycemic loads should be consumed throughout the day, between workouts. Foods with high-glycemic loads—grains and refined sugars, for example—lead to spikes in blood sugar that can cause increased hunger, fatigue, and excessive storage of body fat, besides having low nutrient density.

Glycemic load is a derivative of the glycemic index. The glycemic index measures the effects of the carbohydrate in a particular food on blood sugar levels, based on how quickly they convert to glucose within the human body. The glycemic index uses a numbered scale, with foods higher on the scale causing the quickest increase in blood sugar. Pure glucose and white bread represent the gold standard on this scale, each with a "perfect score" of 100. Peanuts, however, come in with a very low score of 14, as they do not cause much of a blood sugar response. And this makes sense, since peanuts are built more on fat and protein than on carbohydrates, and

converting these to glucose can be the body's equivalent of squeezing water from a stone, so to speak. In general, when considering the glycemic index, we avoid foods that fall much higher than 50 to 55. See glycemicindex.com for a list of common foods and their glycemic index score.

But the glycemic index, while valuable, doesn't really tell us what is happening in the body. Enter the glycemic load. Think of the glycemic index as the theory on which the practicality of the glycemic load is built. While the glycemic index measures the impact the carbohydrate contained in a food has on blood sugar, the glycemic load measures the actual impact of food on blood sugar levels, and it has a scale of 0 to 50. If glycemic load is a book, then glycemic index is its cover. And you know what they say about judging a book.

Let's look at watermelon as an example. The glycemic index of a 100-gram serving of watermelon is quite high, at 72. This number means that the carbohydrate in watermelon would do a nice job of spiking blood sugar. But the glycemic load of the same amount of watermelon is actually very low, at about 3.6—which means that the actual blood sugar response would be minimal. Why is this? Because watermelon contains a ton of water! While the glycemic index of the carbohydrate in watermelon is very high, there is actually very little of it in a typical 100-gram serving. Most of that serving is just water. A 100-gram serving of watermelon contains only about 5 grams of available carbohydrate, because there is so much water.

The glycemic load is calculated by taking a food's glycemic index score, setting it against the "perfect score" of 100, and then multiplying by the amount of carbohydrate in the food. So for a 100-gram serving of watermelon, we set its glycemic index score of 72 against white bread, which is 72/100 = 0.72. We then multiply this number by the serving amount's carbohydrate count, which is 5. So we get 5 × 0.72 = 3.6.

Now, let's look at a different example: spaghetti. Spaghetti has a pretty low glycemic index score of 42. But a single cup of spaghetti contains about 38 grams of carbohydrate. So our equation is (42/100) × 38 = 16. The glycemic load of spaghetti is 16.

Anything having a score of 10 or below is considered pretty low, or light on the blood sugar response; anything at 20 or above is considered high. While the carbohydrate sources in spaghetti have a relatively low impact on blood sugar, spaghetti itself, when eaten in its normal serving size, has a greater impact. So in this sense, it is the opposite of watermelon. On paper, watermelon is a nightmare for blood sugar levels. But in practice, it is about as benign as a food can be. Spaghetti, on the other hand, appears to be pretty benign, but the actuality of it is much greater.

There is one more key element to understanding and using the concept of glycemic load. The first is actual serving sizes versus advertised serving sizes. It's one thing to know the glycemic load of a cup of spaghetti, but I'm sure that I am not the only one who doesn't eat just a single cup of spaghetti when sitting down to dinner. The glycemic load can take this into account as well.

Let's revisit the watermelon example. We discovered that a 100-gram serving of watermelon has a glycemic load score of 3.6, which falls very

QUICK-FIX
SNACKS

The following are a couple of my favorite simple snacks:

1. **A third of a cup of Fruit and Nut Energy Blend** (page 155) is excellent for increasing your intake of essential fatty acids, but don't go overboard! The blend is also high in calories.

2. **An apple or a banana** with 2 tablespoons of peanut butter, almond butter, or sunflower butter.

low on the scale. But what if you had a 200-gram serving? I don't think that I have ever eaten only 100 grams of watermelon. Please! The glycemic index is the same regardless of how much you eat, so it will remain at 72. The remaining variable in the equation is the net carbohydrate count. A 100-gram serving contains about 5 grams of carbohydrate. Therefore, a 200-gram serving contains about 10 grams. So our equation changes: (72/100) × 10 = 7.2. Well, we doubled the serving size, and the glycemic load score doubled, as well. That makes sense. But what does that mean? It means that a 200-gram serving of watermelon will have twice the blood sugar impact of a 100-gram serving. We are putting twice as many carbs into our bodies, and the body is reacting

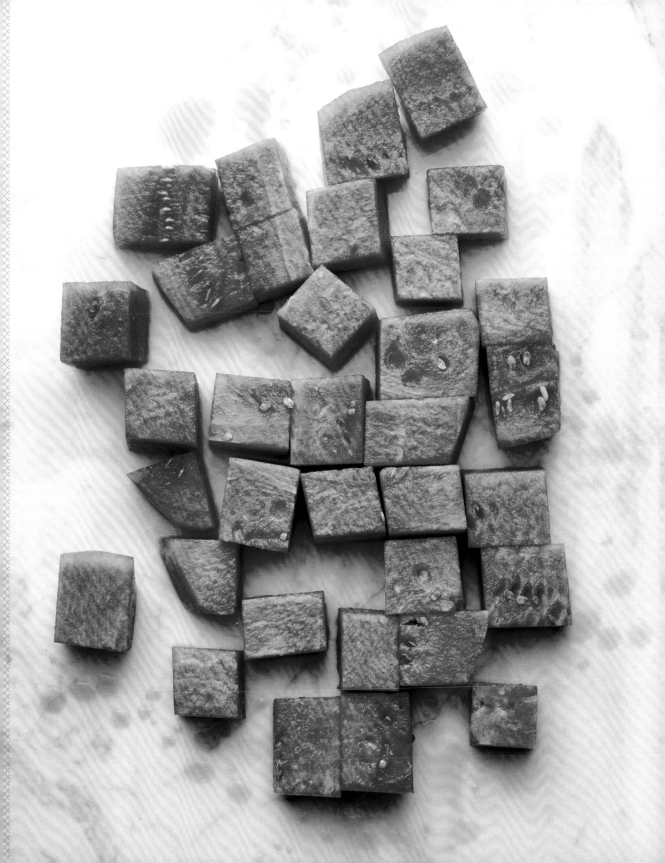

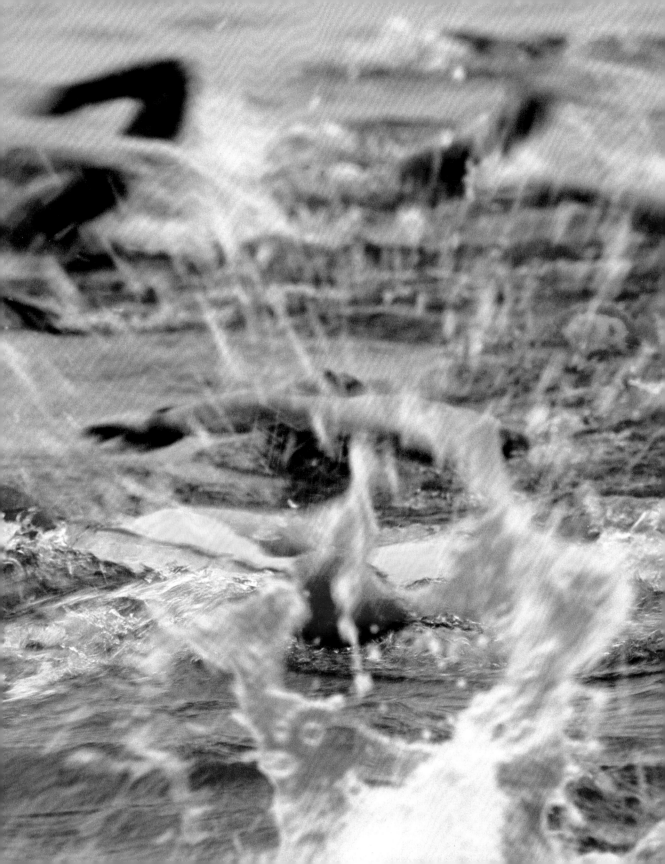

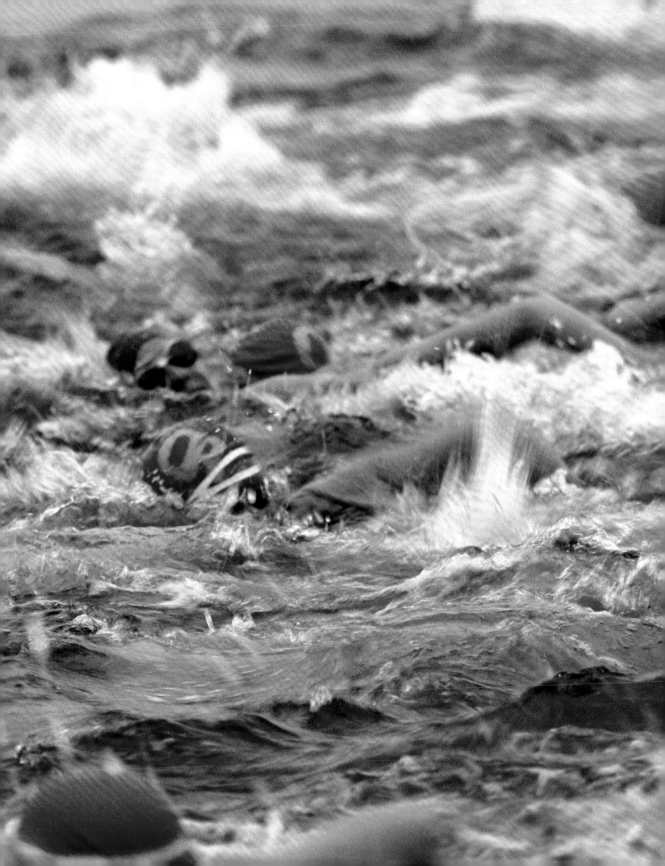

accordingly. Think of it like an 8-ounce glass of water. The glass of water represents the blood in our body, and sweetness represents blood sugar response. The sweeter the water is, the greater the response. If we pour a tablespoon of sugar into the glass, the water becomes sugary. If we pour *two* tablespoons into the glass, it becomes even more sugary. That is exactly what is happening in this watermelon example. The bloodstream gains twice as much carbohydrate when you consume 200 grams of watermelon as when you consume 100 grams of watermelon.

The last important aspect of using glycemic load is considering compound foods. I may have just invented that term, so let me explain. A cheeseburger is a compound food. A turkey sandwich is a compound food. Even pizza is a compound food. Each of these foods is made up of many parts. And most of what we eat every day are compound foods. An apple on its own is clearly a singular item. But when eaten with a bit of peanut butter, it becomes a compound food item. A cheeseburger is made up of the bun, the meat, some cheese, and hopefully some lettuce and tomato. Throw on some ketchup and a little bit of mayonnaise, and we have ourselves a significant blend of different foods. So to understand the impact of the things we eat, we have to look at the entire picture.

Let's take a closer look at a cheeseburger. For the most part, the bun is the only significant source of carbohydrate. The meat, cheese, and condiments are more protein and fat based, which means that while they will change over to blood glucose in time, that conversion will be much more difficult and will not happen

TACKLING A
SWEET TOOTH

To get some antioxidants and avoid too much fat and sugar, while still quenching a sweet craving, try the following:

1. **A square of 70% or higher dark chocolate,** which has more antioxidants and less cocoa fat than chocolate of a lower percentage.

2. **Spread peanut butter on a banana,** and then roll in unsweetened cocoa powder. Freeze until solid.

quickly, so they won't cause much of a spike in blood sugar levels. (The only exception to this is ketchup, which has a fair amount of added sugars.) With low glycemic loads for the meat, cheese, and condiments, and a high glycemic load for the bun, we know what we can cut out to stabilize our blood sugar.

APPLYING GLYCEMIC LOAD
There are two vital ways to apply the concept of glycemic load. The first is to choose foods that have a low glycemic load calculation. Now, I wouldn't try memorizing the specific glycemic load number for every single thing you eat; that would be impractical. Rather, understand the concept and realize that the core foods and approach to fueling

discussed in this book meet the objective. Our goal is to decrease the up-and-down swings that can occur in blood sugar as a result of the foods we eat. By choosing low-glycemic-load foods, we reduce the impact overall, thus stabilizing blood sugar. Core foods—lean meats, lean dairy, fruits, vegetables, nuts, seeds, and legumes—have low glycemic loads, so if you manage to consume just these food types, then you're good to go.

The second application is to eat frequently. The main purpose of eating often is to keep blood sugar levels consistent. We want the body perpetually working to build and rebuild itself so that we can push harder and do better in training, and so that by the time we reach race day, the body is a well-oiled machine. Eating frequently keeps the fires burning, and gives us other benefits, too.

More snacks means more opportunities to put good stuff in your body. Our bodies are working through many macronutrients and micronutrients every hour, and providing new supplies of nutrients often means that you won't run out of fuel—and things like muscle regeneration won't be delayed for lack of the nutrients that keep the process humming.

Consistent intake means your body won't go into fasting mode. When the body isn't sure when food is coming next, it fasts, shifting its focus from burning energy (i.e., the food we ate) to storing it as fat. The point of this is so that we can survive perhaps a long period of time without food. Blame it on thousands of years of evolution; our ancestors really lived that way! We don't need to add pounds of fat when we're gearing up for a race, since it will slow us down. Instead, we need to reassure the body that there will be a steady influx of food and nutrition, so that it can trust us and feel comfortable using our energy intake for energy expenditure versus storing it for later.

Staving off intense hunger will help you stick to your healthy diet. Many times, when hunger rears its head, we either reach for the first thing to eat, no matter what it is, or go overboard and eat way too much. Keep it steady and don't get too hungry, and you'll make good food choices.

Try not to go more than 2 to 3 hours without a snack. For many, this may sound crazy, and it may take time to adjust to the feeling that you're eating all the time—that can be unnerving or annoying to people! Don't panic that you'll gain weight from all of this snacking; if you do it smartly, you'll reap great rewards. Plan to have good food—core foods—with you during the day (stashing healthy bites in your drawers at work is a good thing!). And if you have to rely on purchasing a snack somewhere, remember the core ratio (see page 20).

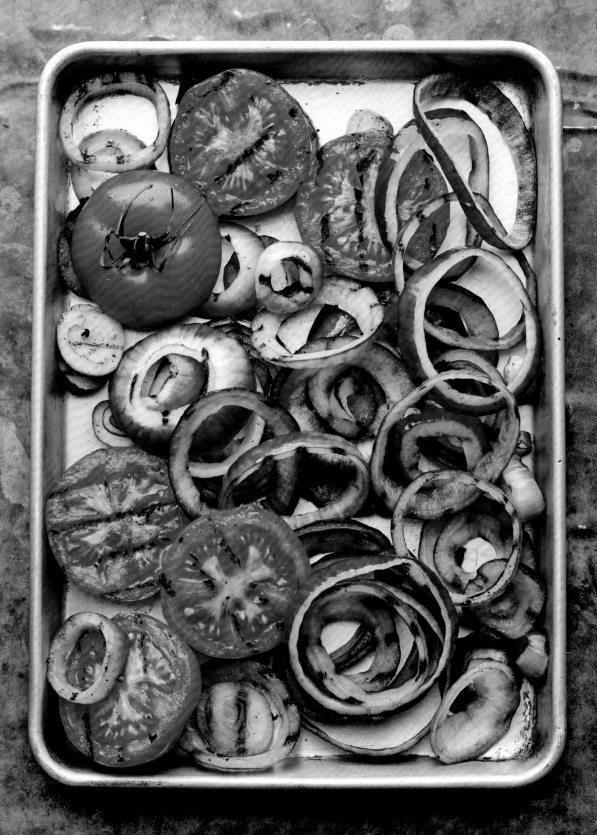

EATING
FOR THE
ATHLETE

3

NOW THAT WE'VE LOOKED CLOSELY AT NUTRITION and how it can affect athletes, let's look at how we can practically use the information to reap benefits during training and racing. How you apply the principles of fueling, in tandem with your workouts, will help you gain the competitive edge that you are hoping for.

THE FUELING WINDOWS

I like to consider three windows of fueling—times designated for taking in nutrition—around training, and then handle racing separately (see page 70). During a training cycle, you'll want to pay close attention to what you consume during these windows: preworkout, during your workout, and postworkout. We'll also look at incorporating a recovery meal, as needed. Workouts should generally be well fueled in order to (1) train the athlete to handle what his or her body requires on race day and (2) ensure that muscle glycogen stays "topped off" for subsequent workout sessions within a training week.

As we know already, grains (like rice, pasta, and bread) and refined sugars should be avoided at any time during the day between workouts because of their lack of nutrients and high impact on blood sugar. But some workout windows can take advantage of these food items, since the

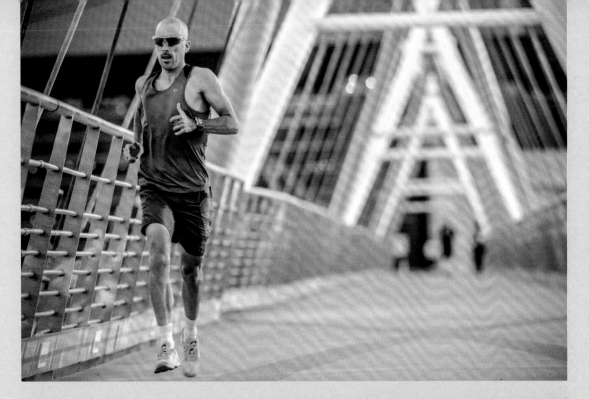

FUELING WINDOWS

WINDOW	EXPLANATION	RECOMMENDATION	CARBOHYDRATE EXAMPLES
Preworkout	Within 1 hour prior to a workout	Easily digestible carbohydrates that are low in fat and fiber	Fig Newtons, gels, bread (waffles, toast, etc.), PowerBar, Nature Valley Granola Bar
During Workout	During the training session itself	Performance fuels that are easily digestible and low in fat and fiber	PowerBar, PowerGel, sports drinks
Recovery Drink	Within ½ hour following a workout	High-glycemic liquids with a 3-to-1 or 4-to-1 ratio of carbohydrate to protein	Klean Recovery drink, or other recovery fuel
Postworkout*	Within a window equal to the workout time following the workout	Moderate-glycemic carbohydrates and a protein source	Whole grains, potatoes, Ezekiel bread, quinoa, oatmeal

The postworkout window changes throughout the year based on your body composition objectives. See page 64 for information on how to manipulate it to reach your goals.

blood sugar response they prompt can be used to help fuel a workout. During these periods, we aren't as focused on nutrient density, because we're more concerned with fueling the workout ahead and not having a nutritionally limited workout session. Some grains and refined sugars are actually good immediate fuel for specific purposes. The table on page 53 shows the windows I generally use, as they relate to workout sessions.

Breads, pastas, sports bars, gels, and sports drinks have a specific purpose for athletes who are looking to get the most out of their training and racing. Used just before, during, or after workouts, these noncore foods will facilitate an increased blood sugar response from the body—and in these cases, we actually *do* want such a response, since it will provide a steady stream of glycogen back to the muscles. That glycogen will enhance the training sessions by (1) giving the muscles the fuel to endure the workload and (2) kick-starting

the recovery process. As they say, "Fat burns in a carbohydrate fire." Carbohydrates consumed before and during workout sessions allow us to apply a greater workload, which in turn burns more calories and fat over the long haul.

PREWORKOUT WINDOW

The purpose of the preworkout window is to start getting blood sugar up to fuel the impending session. You should consume easily digestible carbohydrates to bump up the blood sugar, while including sodium to anticipate loss through sweat. Do not be particularly concerned with nutrient density during this time period. Grains and sugars are perfectly fine, and actually preferred, sources. Always limit fats, fibers, and proteins during this period, as they slow down digestion and therefore can create stomach distress. The amount of carbohydrate should be between 20 and 100 grams, depending on how hungry

PREWORKOUT WINDOW

	LAST REAL SOLID MEAL	LAST LIGHT SOLID FOOD (<50 grams of carbs; minimal protein, fiber, and fat) *	1 GEL PACKET, OR 20 TO 25 GRAMS OF ANOTHER CARBOHY- DRATE FOOD ITEM THAT IS LOW IN PROTEIN, FIBER, AND FAT
Swim	>2 hours	>½ hour	15 minutes
Run	>3 hours	>1 hour	15 minutes
Bike	>1 hour	>½ hour	15 minutes

* Examples include half of a PowerBar, a small bag of pretzels, or four Fig Newtons. Also, check out the recipe section that begins on page 94 for great homemade options for this window.

you are and how long the workout will be. This meal shouldn't weigh you down or aggravate your digestive system. The table on the opposite page gives the time period that I suggest you ideally leave between your last meals and your workouts.

DURING-WORKOUT WINDOW

During workouts, we look to try out and/or replicate what will be our race fueling plans (see page 70). The primary purpose of training nutrition is to train your system to handle the large amounts of nutrition that you'll need during races, and to supply your body with adequate nutrition in order to properly push your body beyond previous training limiters. I generally recommend that athletes consume at least 0.6 gram of carbohydrate per hour per pound of body weight on the bike, and half of that during swimming and running (these are very close to race-day needs, if not the same). For a 150-pound man, this works out to about one gel, half of a bar, or three chew blocks per 30 minutes, plus one bottle of sports drink per hour. For a 120-pound woman, this typically works out to about one gel, half of a bar, or three blocks per 45 minutes, plus one bottle of sports drink per hour. The sodium content of these fuels should be at least 8 to 10 milligrams per gram of carbohydrate, which is consistent with most athletes' minimum sodium needs. Also, try to keep fat and protein content in these fuels to a minimum, unless your workout will be longer than 5 hours. During these longer sessions, it becomes worthwhile to include fat and protein in small quantities. Further, in order to avoid GI distress, keep fiber content as low as practical.

One trick I use with many athletes is ramping up the training fuels to 25% beyond what is planned for race day during the final 10 days before a race (particularly if they'll be racing in hot climates). This acclimates athletes to handle more than they expect to take in on race day, and therefore makes the race-day fuels easier to accept. The funny thing is that most athletes do this totally backward, suddenly trying to ramp up their intake on race day either up to or beyond what they do in training—all while under larger stress and heat on race day! No wonder so many athletes can't handle it and throw up or have a stomach issue.

RECOVERY DRINK

The purpose of a recovery drink is first to replace muscle glycogen as rapidly as possible, and then to provide protein to facilitate muscle synthesis. Because of this, when considering a recovery drink, aim for something that contains a high-glycemic sugar source and a good-quality, easily digested protein, with a carbohydrate-to-protein ratio of 3 to 1 or 4 to 1.

Recovery fuels should be viewed much like training fuels, but with even greater potency. Training fuels typically contain sugar sources that are lower to moderately glycemic in order to spike the blood sugar levels, but at a steady rate. Sources such as sucrose, maltodextrin, brown rice syrup, and fructose all do a nice job of keeping an appropriate stream of glycogen in the blood stream for muscle use. They are flammable, so to speak, but not highly so. Recovery drinks, on the other hand, should be as flammable as possible,

A STUDY OF
STORE-BOUGHT FUELS

These days, there are dozens of good quality foods and drinks on the market and readily available in stores that will fuel our workouts or racing well. Unfortunately, though, plenty of options are inadequate. Here is my review of what's out there—the qualities I look for and some of my favorite products that fit the bill.

DRINKS

For beverages consumed during training sessions, focus on three simple things: carbohydrates, sodium, and quantity of fluid. That's it. Keep it simple! I generally like to have athletes opt for drinks that contain an adequate amount of sodium and about 6 to 7% solution of carbohydrate. That is, a typical 24-ounce bottle of sports drink should contain about 500 to 600 milligrams of sodium and about 40 to 52 grams of carbohydrate. My top choice of sports drinks is Hydro by Base Performance, with Gatorade Endurance and PowerBar Perform coming in as my next preferred options. I like to avoid drinks that contain artificial sweeteners, proteins, vitamins, or minerals. For those of you who would like to take a more natural approach to your sports drink, I've also included a recipe for a homemade version on page 121.

GELS

Tons of gels have come out over the past 10 to 20 years. The early versions had far too little sodium. PowerGel was one of the first to address

this and add more sodium, essentially doubling the amount that others on the market at that time contained. PowerGel is my preferred choice, not only because it has so much more sodium but also because it has a diverse and varied carbohydrate blend, and it leaves out the things you don't need on race day like vitamins or artificial sugars.

One of the most common questions I get about gels and taking gels along with a sports drink is, "Shouldn't I consume this with eight ounces of water, since it says to do so right on the package?" If you look at the carbohydrate solution created by one gel serving and 8 ounces of water, it's about 10 to 12%. As mentioned earlier, the carbohydrate solution of most sports drinks is much lower, at 6 to 7%. If you had only 8 ounces of water for every gel you took on the race course, you'd be fine. The trouble is that most athletes need 24 to 50 ounces of fluid sports drink per hour, and only about one to two gels per hour. With this consumption, it ends up working out to about the same solution of 10 to 12% for a person with a normal sweat rate. I recommend taking gels with sports drinks in training and on race day, which trains your stomach to handle the necessary carbohydrate solution.

BARS

The best bars for training and racing are those that are very low in fat and fiber. This immediately excludes many of the popular bars on the market. PowerBar is a great example of a bar that is low in fat and fiber, as well as diverse in its carb source, and contains moderate protein. Generally, athletes don't need protein on race day unless the duration runs longer than 5 to 6 hours. At that point, it's worth adding a bit of protein—to the tune of about 10 grams per 5 hours of racing. PowerBars are a great option for such scenarios, and they also provide a good amount of sodium. For those who want to take a natural approach with bars during the off season, try the bar and bread recipes in the Natural Workout Fueling section on page 118.

CHEWS

A few companies these days carry chews, and they vary quite a bit in terms of carbohydrate source and sodium content. Clif Bloks are my favorite of the bunch because they have the highest amount of sodium of those I've found, and are sweetened with brown rice syrup, which is an excellent fuel for endurance athletes. Clif also has versions with and without caffeine that are good options.

CARBOHYDRATE CONSUMPTION RECOVERY DRINK (160-POUND MALE)

	LESS THAN 60 MINUTES	GREATER THAN 60 MINUTES OR LESS THAN 70 MINUTES WITH BEST-EFFORT INTENSITY	GREATER THAN 120 MINUTES OR GREATER THAN 70 MINUTES WITH BEST-EFFORT INTENSITY	GREATER THAN 180 MINUTES OR GREATER THAN 120 MINUTES WITH BEST-EFFORT INTENSITY
Swim	None	50 grams	50 grams	N/A
Run	25 grams	50 grams	75 grams	100 grams
Bike	25 grams	50 grams	75 grams	75 grams

from a carbohydrate standpoint. Aim for recovery drinks that use sugar sources such as dextrose, which is an extremely high-glycemic source. But why do we want such a high-glycemic sugar source, if it is the opposite of what we have been preaching throughout all of the previous pages?

Postworkout recovery is a critical time for the muscles of any athlete. After a workout, it is a mad dash to replenish muscle glycogen as quickly as possible. To this end, we want a sugar source that will enter the bloodstream and convert to muscle glycogen at a high rate. Dextrose does exactly this. This is not when we want to maintain a nice stable blood sugar level. Just the opposite, this is when we want blood sugar levels spiked so that the body can shuttle the new glycogen into the empty stores of exercised muscles. The weary muscles quickly recognize this as critical and absorb it accordingly. The correct dosing of recovery drinks replaces about one quarter of the caloric deficit created by the workout. This typically equates to 50 to 100 grams of carbohydrate and 10 to 25 grams of protein. This fueling opportunity will have the single largest impact on your *next* workout. Be sure to have it immediately following your training session.

You may be wondering why protein should be involved if we are so focused on restoring glycogen to the muscles. Protein is essential to a worthwhile recovery drink, because it is what will promote lean muscle repair, fixing the damage that was done during exercise. To this end, whey protein is the finest source, as it is the most effective in this endeavor. Other proteins will help recovery, but they won't necessarily be the most efficient.

The table above gives appropriate amounts of carbohydrate for a 160-pound man to consume, depending upon the nature of a given workout. (These amounts can be loosely scaled, up or down, based on your size. For instance, a 130-pound female would subtract about 25 grams from these values.)

Like most things in life, recovery drinks really are not "one size fits all." In general, I assign athletes a carbohydrate-to-protein ratio of 4 to 1 for optimal recovery. While this is pretty accurate for most people, sometimes other ratios are better.

Athletes who carry too little muscle mass and are focused on gaining strength may want to use a recovery drink that contains a much lower carbohydrate-to-protein ratio, to the tune of 2 to 1 or 3 to 1. These athletes need all the help that they can get in creating an environment that is conducive to muscle development. In addition to a day-to-day diet that focuses on heavy protein intake, their recovery fuels should also have additional proteins. Many endurance athletes either are runners or come from a running background. As you know, runners tend not to be bursting out of the seams of their shirts. They are typically slighter than your average individual, and struggle to build and maintain lean muscle mass. These athletes are prime candidates for a protein-heavy recovery drink, as it will give them an added platform on which to repair, and possibly build, lean muscle mass.

PROTEIN SHAKES
FOR RECOVERY?

If you grew up during the 1990s, you may be scratching your head, wondering what all of this talk about carbohydrates is with regard to muscle recovery. For a long time it was believed that muscle recovery came from protein. Athletes would drink heavy, dense shakes containing upward of 40 grams of protein, with very little carbohydrate. But as it turns out, research has shown that nearly regardless of what kind of exercise you're doing, a combination of carbohydrate and protein, with a heavy concentration on the former, truly promotes muscle recovery.

Even exercises as straightforward as lifting weights require a great amount of muscle glycogen. If a muscle is being worked, then it is likely to be using the glycogen stored in it to do the job. Just like a car, if you want it to run, you need to replenish the fuel, first and foremost. The same is true of our muscles, and carbohydrates supply the fuel they need.

Protein, on the other hand, plays a much lesser role in fueling the muscle, though it does help repair the muscle. Anytime we put stress on the muscles, we damage them. Going back to the car analogy, whereas the carbohydrate acts as the gasoline, the protein works as the auto body repairer after we have been in a fender bender. And endurance athletes get in fender benders almost every day. Just as the auto body repairer makes our car look nice, and therefore run smoothly, without dragging a bumper down the road, the protein helps to repair the damage done to our muscles at the cellular level, so that they can fully recover and run nicely as often as we need them to.

On the flip side of this coin, athletes who carry large amounts of lean muscle mass may want to use a recovery drink that contains a much higher carbohydrate-to-protein ratio, as much as 5 to 1 or even 7 to 1, so that they don't encourage further muscle development. Athletes who carry around a lot of muscle mass may do so to the detriment of their performance. All sports have a certain amount of muscle mass required to not have strength be a limiter. Athletes who are below this level are limited by strength and therefore need to protect and rebuild muscle any time they can. If they are above their sport's level, they can likely lose muscle to improve performance. In these cases, we are much less concerned with protecting and repairing the lean muscle damaged during exercise. The loss of a bit of muscle may be beneficial from a performance standpoint in these cases. A higher ratio allows for a sort of "muscle stripping" to occur. And with the loss of muscle comes the loss of some body weight that may be holding the athlete back. Each pound of unnecessary weight lost can result in a 0.42% increase in performance in biking and 0.62% in running. Note, though, that no more than 1% of the endurance sport population needs to engage in muscle stripping, and it should never be done without the help of a registered dietitian. Having said that, those who are carrying around some extra muscle bulk may want to consider a recovery fuel source that is beyond the general 4 to 1 ratio.

POSTWORKOUT WINDOW

After the recovery drink comes the postworkout window. I define this as an amount of time that follows a session that is as long as the workout was, and it's a time to continue consuming grains and/or refined sugars—fuels that can be immediately put to use for recovery. Here's the logic. During your workouts, you consume enough fuel to replace about half of the expenditure (if you do a good job fueling). Another quarter of that deficit is replaced with the postworkout recovery drink. That leaves about one quarter of the deficit left to replenish. The longer the workout was, the more significant this deficit is, and the more time you need to replace it. The goal of this window is to accomplish a continued rapid replenishment of carbohydrates (and therefore muscle glycogen). Food items that are best to consume during this window include core foods for nutrient density, but with some added grains you typically wouldn't have. For instance, you may have a wrap, or a piece of bread with your protein and veggies. The key is that during this period, your body is still a bit more sensitive to higher-glycemic carbohydrates, using them to replenish what was used during the workout just completed. Later on in the season, this window may be used for whole grains such as oatmeal or whole-grain bread.

This is also the window to manipulate throughout the year to attain body composition objectives. See page 64 for more information.

REPLENISHMENT MEALS

Athletes who train countless hours for endurance events typically fall into a bit of a caloric deficit over the course of the week when following the approach I have outlined in this book. It's important to be careful about deficits, as they can put the body into a weak and vulnerable state. Supplemental fueling by means of gels, sports bars, and sports drinks helps keep glycogen levels up while we are constantly diminishing them, but sometimes these alone are like placing a running garden hose into a large pool of water. A drop in the bucket, so to say. Sometimes the expenditures are just too great to keep up with if we are training very intensely and following a very nutrient-dense, whole-food diet outside our workouts.

Replenishment meals ensure that the race fueling is there—to just top off our store of glycogen and maintain it, given the expenditures during a workout or race day. They ensure that the pool is full. Heavy training and strict adherence to the core foods can slowly begin to drain the glycogen pool, such that the race and training fuels become a heavy percentage of the body's glycogen use. Remember, they are supposed to refill what we use. Therefore, we need to make sure there is something to use in the first place.

A replenishment meal should be heavy in carbohydrates. Remember, we are after the glycogen! Something like a pizza is a great choice—yes, this is license to eat pizza! But not any pizza, since we need to be careful not to include too much saturated fat. So order the pizza. Enjoy the pizza. But cut out the pepperoni. And go light on the cheese. Another example of a replenishment meal is a bowl of pasta with a simple tomato sauce. For the most part, turkey meatballs and bread are nice add-ons. But leave out the sausage. So replenishment meals should have lots of carbohydrates, some protein, and

low amounts of fat (especially saturated fat). And make sure to drink lots of water! In order for the body to properly absorb so many carbs, it needs lots of water or a product such as DRINKmaple, which also contains some electrolytes.

A replenishment meal should be used as a tool, and therefore it should be used at appropriate times. We don't use a hammer when we want to paint a wall, and we don't use a paintbrush when we want to hang a picture. So we need to know when we should be using this tool. Well, when do we want to ensure that we have a full store of glycogen on board? I would argue that we want to be fully stocked in terms of glycogen right before our biggest training day(s) to ensure that they are successful. For many of us, this tends to be on the weekends, but it doesn't have to be. The best rule of thumb is that when we want to make sure that our long workouts are well provisioned, we should incorporate a replenishment meal. For many triathletes, a long ride is typically followed the next day with a long run. This becomes a pretty heavy block of training, over just 2 days. If these workouts occur Saturday and Sunday, then Friday night is the perfect time for a replenishment meal.

The replenishment meal may seem a bit counterintuitive in a book that spends so much time pushing a very whole-foods-oriented diet. But while it can be valuable for an endurance athlete, it isn't always necessary. The point of it is to ward off a caloric deficit, and so those who are not deficient won't need it. A good rule of thumb is that if you are within 85 to 90% compliance with the principles in this book and training heavily as an endurance athlete, then there is a decent chance that you are running at

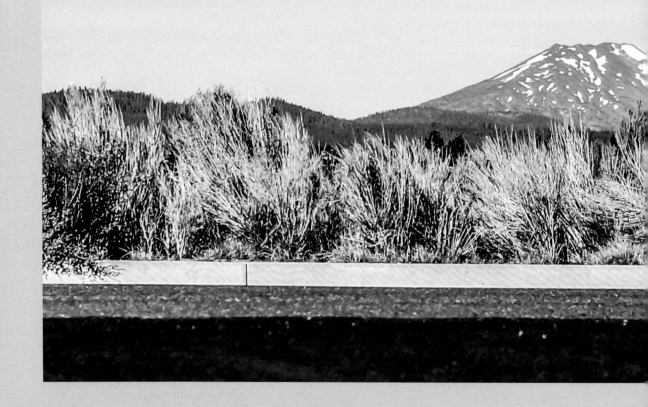

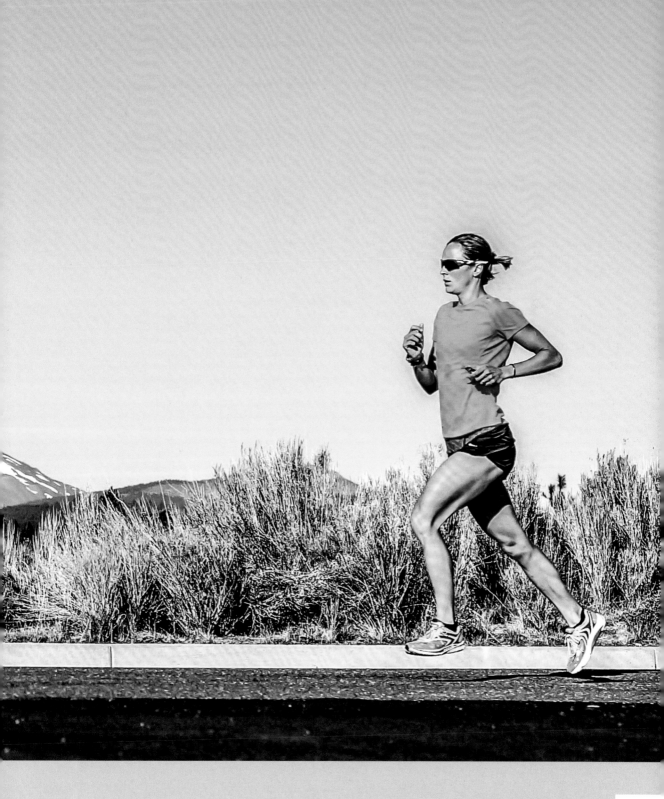

a bit of a deficit. You can also generally know you are running at a deficit by simply noticing how hungry you are. If you feel like you would absorb a loaf of bread on a Friday evening, then you are a prime candidate for a replenishment meal. But if you are not that focused on the principles discussed here, and/or training less than 10 hours per week, then it is quite likely that you are not running much of a deficit, if at all, and the replenishment meal may not be necessary.

BODY COMPOSITION AND NUTRITION PERIODIZATION

Optimizing body composition can be the single easiest thing that athletes can do to improve their performance. Several of the athletes I have worked with went from being a typical age-group triathlete to a professional simply by making changes in the way they eat, which therefore affected body composition. For those of you who run, one pound of unneeded body fat can equal 3 seconds per mile of improved running performance. For those of you who cycle, one pound of unneeded body fat can be worth 1 minute over a 100-mile bike ride. For those of you who swim, there typically isn't much of an impact at all from the loss of body fat. The bottom line is that the impact can be tremendous in most endurance sports, especially when you combine these performance improvements with a better ability to mitigate heat in hot-weather environments.

Nutrition periodization is at the foundation of what I promote in terms of managing nutrition and body composition throughout the year. This concept is about managing what and how much an athlete eats throughout the year to meet specific objectives. In practice, day-to-day eating stays the same throughout the year. Make it a goal to maintain a diet of core foods so that you stock your body with beneficial macronutrients and micronutrients and generally eat healthfully. Then, in racing cycles, you will train your system to be able to handle nutrition when you exercise so that you can handle it on race day, and you never want to have nutritionally limited workout sessions—so you will add the fueling windows to your daily eating. A common error of many athletes (and plenty of nonathletes) is that they try to use workouts to make up for their poor eating earlier in the day and "burn fat" via exercise. What typically happens in these cases is that athletes don't nutritionally prepare for their workout, which in turn doesn't help them train to handle more nutrition during their races, and, worse yet, they end workouts so hungry that they make further mistakes by consuming high-glycemic foods that are void of nutrient density later in the day.

The healthy way to use nutrition periodization to achieve body composition goals is by manipulating the postworkout window. Here is how to adjust it throughout the year:

• During the off-season, use the postworkout window as a chance to have what you want. Many times this means pizza or other noncore foods that actually overshoot the deficit from the workout, creating a caloric surplus, and the athlete gains weight. Adding pounds is a good thing during the off-season when coming from a very lean race weight. I generally like to see athletes gain 6 to 8 pounds from their lean, race-ready body weight during this time of year to promote a full physical and mental recovery! If you are even greater than 8 pounds from your lean race weight, you should remove the post-workout window, which will act as a catalyst for your weight loss via a slight daily caloric deficit.

- Four to 6 months out from a major race or the primary race season, most athletes should begin to stabilize their weight by eating whole grains during the postworkout window. Whole grains provide added carbohydrates to replenish blood sugar, but by focusing on them, you're less likely to overshoot your caloric needs. Whole grains tend to be self-limiting because of the amount of protein and fiber they contain (in other words, they fill you up faster).

- During the final 6 to 8 weeks before your major race or race season, remove the postworkout window to create a caloric deficit and lose weight. This will help trim little bits of unneeded body fat to get you down to race weight.

When you look more closely at how this approach works, you'll see that nutrition periodization takes care of itself. That is, during the off-season when there are fewer training sessions, the preworkout, during-workout, and postworkout windows are all dropped. Then, without these windows, your diet will consist of all core foods, which tend to be rich in fat, fiber, and protein, while lower in carbohydrates. Eating in this fashion can result in a macronutrient profile of 30% carbohydrate, 40% fat, and 30% protein.

Conversely, during race season, with many workouts during the week and the addition of the fueling windows, the macronutrient profile can be as high as 70% carbohydrate, 20% fat, and 10% protein. So using the fueling windows results in following the concept of nutrition periodization.

RACE WEIGHT

Athletes mostly think about body composition in a one-dimensional way, or they don't think about it at all. Most do not get too far beyond considering only their body weight and/or the percentage of their body weight that comes from fat. I'd like to outline a more effective, sport-specific approach to looking at body composition, using traditional metrics in a more synergistic way. The two primary metrics to consider are body fat percentage and body mass index.

Body fat percentage (BF%) is the percentage of your total body weight that is made up of fat. This can be tested roughly with an impedance scale, such as those made by Tanita, or more accurately by getting measured with body fat calipers at your local fitness club.

Body mass index (BMI) indicates how your total body weight compares to your height. You can calculate it by multiplying your body weight (in pounds) by 703, and then dividing that number by your height (in inches) squared.

There is limited sport-specific value in using the metrics of BF% and BMI separately. However, when used in conjunction, they can provide deep insight into sport-related limiters. To do this, I like to consider two types of body composition goals: short term and long term.

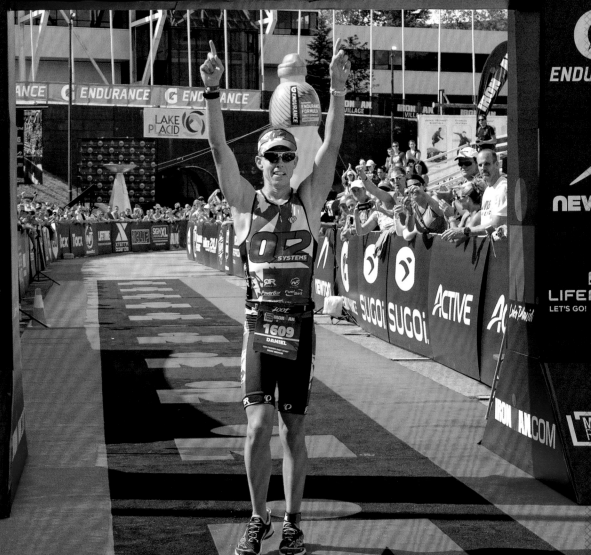

Short-Term Race Weight

Short-term race weight in my mind is about body fat, something we can manipulate fairly easily over weeks or months via dietary changes to reach a certain goal. Many athletes confuse this with overall body weight. I hear people say, "I was 120 pounds when I was twenty-two and a great runner! But now I'm thirty-eight and weigh 135. I need to get back down there!" This creates a dangerously slippery slope where the athlete strives directly for a specific weight without thinking about muscle gained over the period—muscle that may be beneficial for the sport they are now doing! By targeting only a specific weight, they aim for something that could be detrimental to performance and health over the short term. In this example, the 38-year-old person at 135 pounds may have a body fat of 13%. If this is a woman, she probably wouldn't want to go much lower! However, as this person chases a body weight over the short term, not realizing the amount of muscle gained, he or she ends up driving body fat *way* too low to be healthy.

The first step in carrying out a detailed evaluation of body composition is to take an accurate measurement of body fat. There is no need to go crazy in getting an exact number; plus or minus 1.5% will be more than appropriate. Then, work with a dietitian and/or coach to target an approximate race-day BF%. Assuming this percentage is about as low as the athlete should safely be, based on age and gender, a goal body weight should then be determined under the assumption that this goal BF% can be reached via dietary manipulation over the short term. For example, if a male athlete currently weighs 160 pounds with a BF% of 12%, and has an optimal/goal BF% of 8%, we would assume that the athlete will lose 4 percent of his body weight through dietary manipulation. To determine this athlete's goal race-day body weight we calculate 4% of 160 (.04 × 160), which is about 6 pounds. Assuming that this athlete does not lose a significant amount of muscle during the weight loss phase, he can expect to race at about 154 pounds and 8% body fat. This is the athlete's lean adjusted body weight. This process is a powerful tool for helping to determine an athlete's optimal short-term race weight, as well as the impacts on performance that may be seen by reaching this optimal body weight. Assuming that this goal BF% has been properly determined and that there has not been a significant loss of strength due to a loss of lean muscle mass, each pound of lost body weight roughly equates to a 3 seconds/pound/mile improvement in running pace and about 3 seconds/pound for every 4 miles on the bike. With this in mind, once our example athlete has shed those 6 pounds of body fat, he can expect an improvement of about 18 seconds/mile in his run pace and 18 seconds/4 miles in his bike pace.

Long-Term Race Weight

Long-term race weight is much more focused on muscle content goals than on fat. Here, we integrate BMI into the evaluation of an athlete's body composition, alongside BF%, which allows us to consider the athlete's muscle mass content. Let's consider the idea that every sport has its own optimal BMI number, where strength does not act as a limiter to performance and is not in excess of what is needed. If an athlete's lean adjusted body weight results in a BMI that is below the sport's requirement, then there is a good chance that inadequate strength acts as a limiter to his or her performance. In this case, strength should be a primary target of the athlete's training plan, along with the appropriate dietary changes to support muscle mass development. This would mean a greater focus on protein content in the diet, and a significant period of higher body fat each year to support muscle mass development. This also helps provide injury resistance for athletes who are injury prone.

To calculate lean BMI, multiply the lean adjusted body weight in pounds by 703, and then divide this number by the square of the athlete's height in inches. If this lean adjusted BMI is much above that required for the selected sport, then it is likely that the extra muscle mass being carried around is not needed for optimal performance in the sport and actually slows down the athlete. In my experience regarding triathlons, the optimal lean adjusted BMI is about 20 for women and 21 for men. For runners this is about 19 for women and 18 for men. Remember, this metric has value only when combined with BF% to create a lean adjusted body weight for the BMI calculation. For example, if BMI is calculated for an athlete with significant body fat without first being adjusted for lean body weight, it will result in an artificially high number because of significant body fat, with no correlation to the sport-specific strength evaluation. A sport such as rowing would have a higher optimal BMI because of the significant strength component required.

When evaluating the sport-specific body composition of a new athlete, the typical process is to (1) determine her current BF% and, with the assistance of a good coach or dietitian, determine a target race-day BF%; (2) adjust body weight assuming that this goal will be reached; (3) calculate BMI with this lean adjusted body weight; (4) evaluate this BMI versus the aforementioned sport-specific ideals; and (5) if she is above or below these ideals, consider manipulating her training and/or nutrition program, with the goal of working toward these ideals. How to go about reaching these goals in terms of muscle mass gain/loss is beyond the scope of this book, as it can be very specific and quite complicated. Regardless, the process outlined earlier sheds light on how an athlete may be able to squeeze additional speed out of an already sound training program and further understand where her specific limiters may lie. Only when BF% and BMI are combined does a truly powerful tool for evaluating potential athletic limiters become apparent.

FAST RECOVERY BETWEEN EVENTS

From time to time you may be racing on both weekend days, or need to recover very quickly to ensure a smooth and immediate return to the training routine. The following recovery protocol can go a long way in making this possible. I've used this for years!

1. **Less than 30 minutes after the race:** Consume a recovery drink that contains approximately

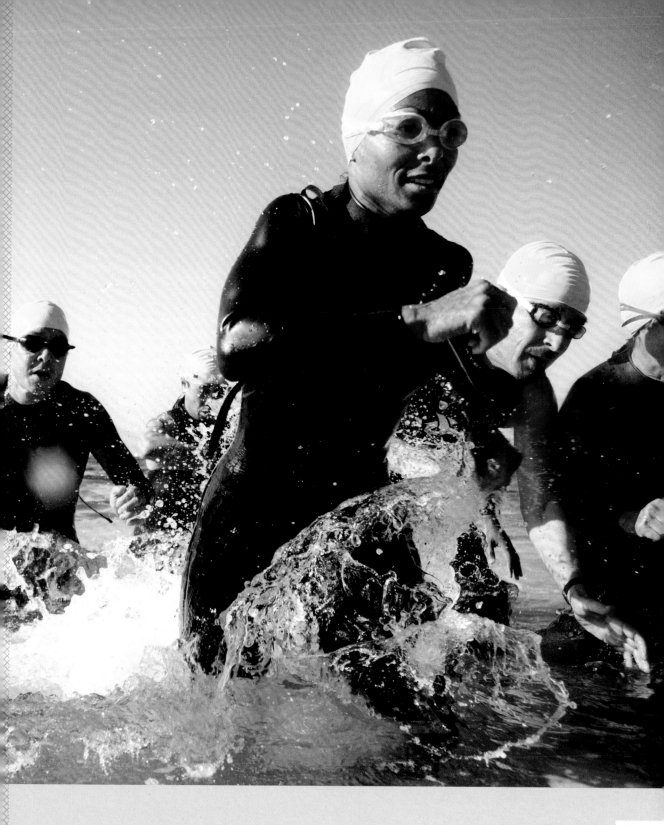

a 4-to-1 ratio of carbohydrates to protein. This drink should also contain at least 5 grams of the amino acid L-glutamine (see page 91). Klean Recovery Drink is a great choice but will require the supplementation of additional L-glutamine.

2. **Thirty to 90 minutes after the race:** Snack on raisins, pretzels, and water. Have enough to feel satisfied but not stuffed.

3. **Two hours after the race:** Have a cinnamon raisin bagel and two scoops of whey protein. Supplement this with 1,000 milligrams of vitamin C and 5,000 milligrams of EPA/DHA from fish oil (see page 91).

4. **Two to 4 hours after the race:** Sip on green tea and snack on pretzels and prunes. Also begin considering a balanced meal of protein and carbohydrate during this period, with two to four servings of fruits and/or vegetables.

The preceding protocol will provide nutrients and antioxidants to support your immune system, as well as facilitate muscle recovery following an intense or long-distance event. Each food choice throughout the 4-hour period has a specific purpose to fuel rapid recovery:

L-GLUTAMINE: This nonessential amino acid is heavily depleted during intense exercise. It is also one of the most abundant amino acids in the muscle cell, and therefore it's beneficial to supplement after a tough race to replenish what was lost; see page 91 for more information.

RAISINS: A very alkaline food, raisins have been theorized to lower blood pH following hard workouts. They are also high-glycemic, which helps restock muscle glycogen.

BAGEL: An easy introduction to eating whole foods, bagels are high-glycemic and contain about 85% carbohydrate for the rapid replenishment of muscle glycogen. They also contain about 10 grams of protein, aiding in the repair of damaged muscle. Cinnamon raisin bagels are the best option, for the benefits of the raisins, as described earlier.

VITAMIN C: A large dose of vitamin C has been shown to boost the immune system and assist in free radical neutralization.

EPA/DHA: Omega-3 fatty acids have been shown to lessen inflammation and can potentially reduce exercise-induced swelling of muscle tissue. See more about omega-3s on page 32, and more on supplements on page 37.

GREEN TEA: Extremely high in antioxidants, green tea has been shown to boost the immune system and assist in free radical neutralization. The antioxidant present in this type of tea is one of the most potent known to humankind: EGCG (epigallocatechin gallate).

RACE-DAY AND DURING-RACE FUELING

Race fueling often becomes the primary limiter for athletes racing longer distances. As an athlete, your objective is to do everything that you can to help reduce this possibility. The sacrifices you make in training are often extreme, with time spent away from family and friends. Nutritionally limited races make these sacrifices feel like they have been made in vain, leaving the athlete with little return on the investment.

The probability that you have fueling limiters on race day is mostly determined by the difference between what your body needs in the form of carbohydrates per hour and what your digestive system can handle. The more you can handle, and the less you need, the larger your fueling insurance policy. The larger the policy, the greater likelihood that poor fueling won't be a limiter for you on race day. The most common issue is that athletes don't eat or drink enough during sessions, and therefore train themselves to handle less and less, thereby reducing the insurance policy.

The major issue associated with consuming too little in training is that over time, these athletes not only train their bodies to use less but also (unintentionally) train the digestive system to handle less. Because the primary limiter for many long-course racers is the ability to handle race nutrition, decreasing one's ability to do so wreaks havoc on race day, thereby preventing the athlete from reaching other limiters, such as fitness itself. Anything we can do to remove the fuel digestion limiter will lead to greater gains than that 1% potential gain in metabolic efficiency espoused by those who promote eating less in training.

The lesson here is that while a low-intake approach in training—maybe even incorporating fasted workouts occasionally—may improve metabolic efficiency and reduce the amount of fuel your body requires many times, the result is

still a net loss in performance due to the inability of the athlete to handle what the body requires, especially in long races. Even if eating less in training gives athletes a slight gain in metabolic efficiency through dietary manipulation, that process narrows their "insurance policy" and reduces their ability to digest and handle nutrition, a key factor in their success.

Instead, if athletes implement robust fueling plans during training sessions, they will widen their fueling insurance policy, preparing the body to handle the quantity and type of fuel necessary to race to their potential. Maximizing that fueling insurance policy creates a more resilient gut, capable of absorbing and digesting the massive quantities of nutrition required to fuel a strong run. To build up the resilience, we must train the gut for peak performance, just as we train our muscles, every day and in every session.

There are a few exceptions. A small percentage of the population will be able to practice the low-intake approach in training and yet not experience gastrointestinal issues on race day. In these cases, the athlete typically was born with an impressive digestive system that handles an inordinate amount of fluids and carbohydrates and generally exhibits lower sweat rates. Also, these athletes are probably completing races that are less than 3 hours long. However, the primary limiter in longer-distance racing is the inability to handle nutrition. Thus, the greatest net gain is achieved in training the gut and widening the fueling insurance policy and not in obtaining a possible metabolic efficiency advantage in early stages of the race that only results in an insurance policy that is so small that the body is unable to

CARB-LOADING EXAMPLES

2 DAYS BEFORE MARATHON

CALORIES: 2,128

TIME	DESCRIPTION	PROTEIN	CARBS	FAT	FIBER
7:00	Scrambled eggs	15 g.	2 g.	5 g.	3 g.
	Banana	1 g.	25 g.	0 g.	3 g.
8:30	3 Fat-free Fig Newtons (or 1 gel)	1.5 g.	33 g.	0 g.	1.5 g.
9:00	S/B/R workout drink (1 bottle)	0 g.	50 g.	0 g.	0 g.
10:15	Klean Recovery Drink (1 scoop)	10 g.	40 g.	0 g.	0 g.
10:30	2% Greek yogurt	17 g.	8 g.	4 g.	0 g.
12:00	Lunch (salad)	15 g.	45 g.	8 g.	0 g.
4:30	Clif Builder's Bar	20 g.	30 g.	8 g.	4 g.
7:00	LARGE dinner!	15 g.	90 g.	15 g.	0 g.
9:00	Protein shake (1 scoop)	18 g.	2 g.	2 g.	0 g.
	TOTAL:	**112.5 G.**	**325 G.**	**42 G.**	**11.5 G.**
	PERCENT:	**21%**	**61%**	**18%**	

1 DAY BEFORE RACE
LONGER THAN 1.5 HOURS

CALORIES: 3,704.5

TIME	DESCRIPTION	PROTEIN	CARBS	FAT	FIBER
8:00	BIG breakfast	20 g.	140 g.	25 g.	0 g.
	Sports drink (1 bike bottle)	0 g.	50 g.	0 g.	0 g.
10:00	Fat-free Fig Newtons x 6	3 g.	66 g.	0 g.	3 g.
12:00	Pretzels (8 oz.) - EAT ALL DAY	24 g.	192 g.	8 g.	8 g.
1:00	Pita, wrap, or bread	6 g.	34 g.	1 g.	1 g.
	Sliced turkey (6 oz.)	36 g.	0 g.	0 g.	0 g.
3:00	PowerBar	10 g.	45 g.	2 g.	3 g.
4:00	Sports drink (1 bike bottle)	0 g.	50 g.	0 g.	3 g.
5:00	Fat-free Fig Newtons x 6	3 g.	66 g.	0 g.	3 g.
7:30	Grilled chicken breast	26 g.	0 g.	3 g.	0 g.
	Small bowl (1.5 cups) of pasta	10 g.	54 g.	1.5 g.	3 g.
	TOTAL:	**138 G.**	**697 G.**	**40.5 G.**	**24 G.**
	PERCENT:	**15%**	**75%**	**10%**	

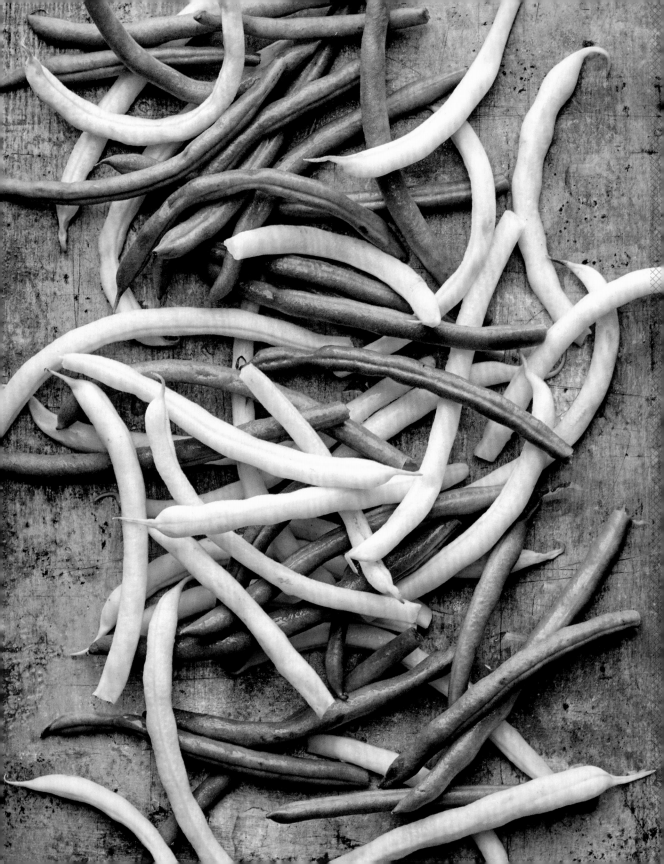

digest even the tiniest amount in the latter stages of the race.

I believe that the lion's share of metabolic efficiency comes from (1) training at proper intensities and (2) day-to-day eating in accordance with the principles in this book. That, combined with fueling the workouts properly with carbohydrates, gets athletes the best of both worlds: their bodies will be metabolically efficient while still able to handle huge amounts of fuels on race day.

The following section outlines the basics of a successful fueling program. The strategy should be planned with the highest regard, as many times fueling habits are what limit the athlete on race day.

CARBOHYDRATE LOADING FOR YOUR EVENT

The carbohydrate load is meant to make sure that your body—in particular, the liver and the muscles—is as full of glycogen as it possibly can be. This gives you a reservoir from which to draw throughout race day. For many athletes, carb loading should begin 2 days before the race around lunchtime or dinnertime, depending on the length of the race. For races under 5 hours, the load can start the day before the race since the carbohydrate load isn't as critical. For races less than 1.5 hours, no carb load is needed at all! The carbohydrate load is typically kicked off by incorporating grains that the athlete would not typically have, but without going overboard. Then the primary loading moment should take place on the day before the event, with breakfast being the largest meal. This breakfast should be completed before nine a.m. at the latest, with the

remainder of the day's food being eaten as very frequent snacks, tapering throughout the day and culminating in a final light meal for dinner. Ideally, 50% of the day's carbs should be consumed by noon. This approach allows for complete glycogen loading, while leaving proper time for digestion before the race starts. The foods you choose for the carb load should be very low in fat and fiber. This is not a time to eat practically *any* fruits and vegetables, since they slow digestion. Having a salad the day before the race will not help you go any faster; it only runs the risk of slowing down digestion and limiting your race. It's the salad you had every day for the past 2 years that helped you absorb more training stress and become faster over the long haul! Eating high-fiber fruits and vegetables during this time frame is a common mistake. A good rule of thumb for the carbohydrate load is to define your carb intake goal for the entire day as follows: consume enough grams of carbohydrate to equal approximately 4.5 times your body weight in pounds. See the tables on pages 72 and 73 for carb load examples.

RACE MORNING

Breakfast on race morning should contain between 110 and 180 grams of carbohydrate, depending on your size and the race distance. A good rule of thumb is to multiply your lean body weight (see page 67) in pounds by 1.2 for IRONMAN-distance triathlons and 1 for Olympic-distance triathlons to get the amount of carbohydrates in grams that you should eat. For runners, a factor of 1 works great for almost all

IRONMAN RACE NUTRITION

	TIME	DESCRIPTION	CARBS (G)	SODIUM (G)
BREAKFAST:	-3:30	3.5 cups applesauce	112	0
		1 banana	25	0
		1 scoop, whey protein	0	60
		1 bottle, sport drink	51	600
PRERACE:	-1:00	1 PowerBar	45	260
	-0:15	PowerGel with 8 ounces water	27	200
RACE:	1:15	½ PowerBar	22.5	130
	1:45	½ PowerBar	22.5	130
	2:15	PowerGel (caffeinated)	27	200
	2:45	PowerGel (caffeinated)	27	200
	3:15	PowerGel (caffeinated)	27	200
	3:45	½ PowerBar	22.5	130
	4:15	½ PowerBar	22.5	130
	4:45	Power Gel (caffeinated)	27	200
	5:15	Power Gel (caffeinated)	27	200
	5:45	Power Gel (caffeinated)	27	200
	6:15	Power Gel (caffeinated)	27	200
	6:45	Power Gel (caffeinated)	27	200
	7:15	banana	25	0
		7 bottles, Hydro Sports Drink (over the course of the bike)	357	4,200
	9:00	Clif Bloks	48	140
		PowerGel (caffeinated)	27	200
	11:00	Clif Bloks (caffeinated)	48	140
		PowerGel (caffeinated)	27	200
		PowerGel (caffeinated)	27	200
		TOTAL:	937	8,320
		QUANTITY PER HOUR:	85	756

NOTES:

1 The total carb count does not include breakfast or prerace intake. However, the total sodium count includes all intake. The quantity per hour for carbs and sodium includes only during-race intake.

2 Drink about 4 ounces of sport drink (if you can), or water at each aid station during the run.

3 In an IRONMAN, 1 Clif Blok should be eaten every 2 miles of the run.

4 Applesauce should be unsweetened.

5 Only use caffeine and caffeinated supplements where indicated— and if you have trained with them and are comfortable taking them.

6 When the weather is warmer than 80 to 85°F., make sure you get ahead with sports drink early on the bike.

½ IRONMAN RACE NUTRITION

	TIME	DESCRIPTION	CARBS (G)	SODIUM (G)
BREAKFAST:	-3:00	2.75 cups applesauce	88	0
		1 banana	25	0
		1 scoop, whey protein	0	60
		1 bottle, sports drink	51	600
PRERACE:	-0:15	PowerGel (caffeinated) with 8 ounces water	27	200
RACE:	0:40	½ PowerBar	22.5	130
	1:20	PowerGel (caffeinated)	27	200
	2:00	PowerGel (caffeinated)	27	200
	2:40	3 Clif Bloks (caffeinated)	24	70
	3:20	3 Clif Bloks (caffeinated)	24	70
		3.5 bottles, Hydro Sports Drink (over the course of the bike)	179	2,100
	4:05	PowerGel (caffeinated)	27	200
		TOTAL:	357	3,830
		QUANTITY PER HOUR:	71	540

MARATHON RACE NUTRITION

	TIME	DESCRIPTION	CARBS (G)	SODIUM (G)
BREAKFAST:	-3:00	2.75 cups applesauce	88	0
		1 banana	25	0
		1 scoop, whey protein	0	60
		1 bottle, sports drink	51	600
PRERACE:	-0:30	100 mg. caffeine		
	-0:15	PowerGel (caffeinated) with 8 ounces water	27	200
RACE:	0:30	PowerGel	27	200
	1:00	PowerGel (caffeinated)	27	200
	1:30	PowerGel (caffeinated)	27	200
	2:00	PowerGel (caffeinated)	27	200
	2:30	PowerGel (caffeinated)	27	200
		TOTAL:	162	1,860
		QUANTITY PER HOUR:	46	531

distances from 5K to marathon. Again, go very light on fat or fiber here, if you include any at all, to avoid a delay in digestion. As an example, a good option would be 2.5 cups of unsweetened applesauce, one scoop of whey protein, one bottle of a sports drink, and a banana. This breakfast should be consumed about 3.5 hours before the start of IRONMAN-distance triathlons, 3 hours before half-IRONMAN-distance triathlons or marathons, and 2.5 hours before Olympic-distance triathlons or half marathons. Other sports can be related to these guidelines simply by the duration of their events.

DURING RACING

Your body will need lots of fluids, as well as lots of carbohydrates during the race itself. Racing nutrition is primarily about providing the fluid your body needs so that it doesn't exceed a 2% dehydrated state. That is, you should never lose more than 2% of your body weight during training or racing, since this is the threshold where performance is affected. If you manage this, along with getting the levels of sodium you require, you've solved 90% of the issues athletes have on race day!

Fluids

Although there are several ways for you to determine your sweat rate, I like to keep it as simple as possible. Aim to urinate at least twice during the bike portion of a full IRONMAN-distance triathlon, and at least once during the bike portion of a half-IRONMAN-distance triathlon. Athletes who fail to do this will not

typically run to their potential. More detailed sweat testing can certainly be completed, but this is by far the easiest and often most effective way to evaluate your sweat rate. The key is to drink enough to make sure you urinate at these rates. Think back to some of your prior race experiences, what the weather was, how much you drank, and how many times you peed. Most athletes can get a very good idea of their fluid requirements by doing this exercise.

For shorter triathlon race distances and for running races, you may not pee at all. In these cases, it's worth doing a simple test by weighing yourself before and after a 30-minute to 1-hour bike or run that is completed in conditions similar to those expected on race day. To do the test properly, try to pace it similar to the pace of race day, and keep track of anything that you drink during the session. You can then take the difference between the before and after weights in pounds and multiply it by 16 ounces. This is the amount of fluid lost (and not replaced) from your body during the session itself. Add to that the amount you drank, and you have the amount of sweat loss. This amount of sweat loss can be converted to the hourly fluid losses by dividing 60 by the duration of the session in minutes and multiplying it times the fluid loss in ounces. Any race where you lose more than 2% of body weight (3 pounds for a 150-pound individual) is a race where your performance will be limited. Armed with this information and the sweat test fluid losses, you can figure out your fluid requirements for race day. For instance, if you weigh 150 pounds and plan to do a 2-hour race, you can lose up to 3 pounds over the course of the event. That translates to 48 ounces of fluids. If your sweat test determined that your losses will be 50 ounces per hour, you only need to drink 26 ounces per hour on race day.

Carbohydrates

Carbohydrate intake for most triathlon races should be approximately 0.64 gram for each pound of lean body weight. For example, this would be about 96 grams per hour for a 160-pound athlete at 6% BF. For Olympic-distance and sprint-distance triathlons, this value can be as low as 0.5 gram per pound. This calculation estimates the average carbohydrate need over the entire triathlon race, including intake during both the bike and run portions of the event. For most athletes, the run intake should be about two thirds of this average per hour, and therefore a bit higher on the bike. For running-only races, this intake is about 0.3 gram of carbs per pound of lean body weight.

Most research—and practical feedback—shows that varying the source of carbohydrate is a good approach on race day—that is, using products that blend the use of higher- and lower-glycemic sources of carbohydrate. How an athlete gets the required amount of carbohydrate is more a matter of preference and convenience than anything else. There is significant value in keeping things simple, so look for products that contain varying types of carbohydrates, with adequate sodium, to keep the plan simple and easy to execute on race day. Similarly, avoiding products that contain significant sources of fat, protein, or fiber is a good approach, especially for those who have experienced stomach distress in prior races.

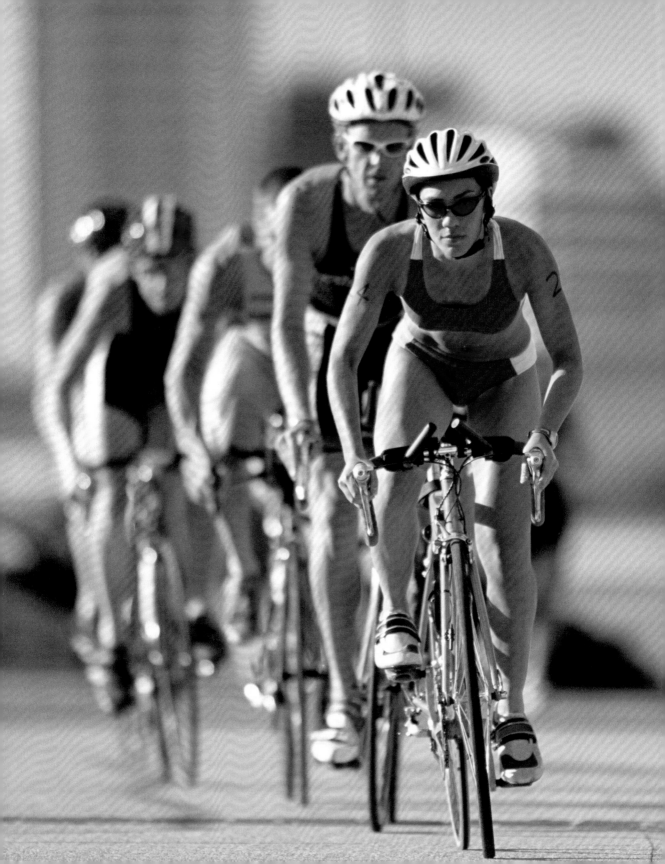

STRESS, THE TRIADS, AND GI HEALTH

NOW THAT WE HAVE COVERED the nuts and bolts, from how to eat during the day to fueling during your workouts and racing, I'll cover some additional concepts that are important to nutrition as it relates to athletics.

STRESS AND THE FEMALE ATHLETE TRIAD

Most athletes have heard of the female athlete triad. It is a combination of three conditions—disordered eating, amenorrhea, and osteoporosis—that all develop out of stress due to high training and inadequate nutrient intake. Endurance sports should be approached with a total stress budget in mind, meaning you should take all of the following into account to manage the stress you're enduring:

1. **Enhance restorative techniques** to increase the capacity for added stress. Specifically, work on getting good-quality sleep and maintaining good-quality nutrition.
2. **Maximize the amount of good stress** applied. Good stress, in this case, is exercise.
3. **Minimize the amount of bad stress**—such as work stress, poor nutrition, and drugs.

Regardless of the type of stress, all athletes have a total stress budget available to spend. We want to fill it with as much good stress as we can, minimize bad stress expenditures, and enhance the budget with good restorative techniques. The female athlete triad occurs when the budget is exceeded.

DISORDERED EATING

The primary cause of the female athlete triad is disordered eating and the resulting impact on caloric, vitamin, and mineral intake. For athletes, this disordered eating is fueled by the perception that thinner is always better. I can tell you that it certainly isn't; there's absolutely a point for every person where thin is too thin. Many times, in the attempt to lose weight for racing purposes, athletes develop more serious eating disorders such as anorexia or bulimia.

AMENORRHEA

Irregular menstrual cycles are also a factor in the female athlete triad. Amenorrhea, which is defined as a lack of a menstrual period for 3 months in a row, is quite common among female triathletes and marathon runners. However, those who struggle with disordered eating have an elevated risk of developing amenorrhea. One impact of the lack of a menstrual cycle in female athletes is its impact on estrogen, one of the most important female hormones. The lack of a cycle generally results in lower levels of estrogen, which in turn negatively impacts bone strength and leads to the next aspect of the female athlete triad: osteoporosis.

OSTEOPOROSIS

Women with the female athlete triad have a higher risk of developing osteoporosis as a result of low nutrient intake due to disordered eating in combination with the stress of high levels of training. Osteoporosis occurs when bones lose mass, weaken, and become brittle, and those with this condition will get stress fractures more easily and frequently. The triad includes osteoporosis because the lack of nutrient intake related to the disordered eating and the lack of estrogen from amenorrhea result in decreased bone mass.

WHAT TO WATCH OUT FOR

Here is a checklist for female athletes who worry they may have developed, or may be developing, the female athlete triad:

1. Do you find yourself being very restrictive with your dietary intake even when others (like coaches and dietitians) say that you shouldn't be?
2. Have you had more than one stress fracture within the past 2 years?
3. Have you not had a menstrual cycle in the past 90 days?
4. Do you try to stay lean year-round, even when not in the competitive season?
5. Do you experience extreme fatigue and/or low self-esteem or depression?

If you answered "yes" to at least three of the preceding questions, there is a good chance you

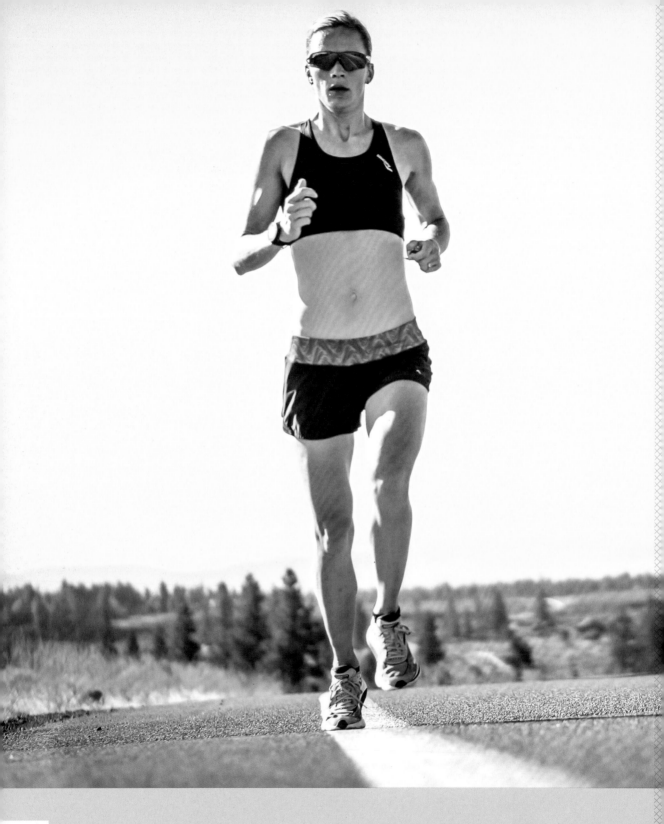

may have or be on the path to the female athlete triad. If so, you should work with a coach and/or psychologist to discuss your mental health, and work closely with a dietitian to establish a support of healthy nutrition habits.

THE ENDURANCE ATHLETE TRIAD

Although the female athlete triad is a well-known medical issue, I've witnessed a much less severe and performance-based type of acute triad that can plague athletes, male or female, beginner or professional. I call it the endurance athlete triad, and while it's more dangerous at longer racing distances, it can undermine potentially great performances at all race lengths. The endurance athlete triad is defined by three factors: (1) a weak state of mental fitness (self-imposed pressures), (2) overdoing workout intensity, and (3) overdieting. Athletes with this condition often show up on race day with a mental atmosphere lacking any sense of confidence and a body that is malnourished and overtired. It typically results in a disappointing finish, which further feeds into an already present lack of confidence, pushing the athlete into a downward spiral of negativity. Among athletes with a type A personality, the usual response is to work harder and place even more dietary restrictions on oneself. This is a certain recipe for disaster! In females, chronic occurrence of the endurance athlete triad can certainly lead to the female athlete triad, as the root causes follow similar psychological patterns.

Here's an example of the endurance athlete triad. Not too long ago, I was working with Jane (not her real name), an age-group athlete who fell into the preceding scenario. She was training for a marathon, with the ultimate goal of qualifying for Boston. Early on in training, she heard everything I had to say regarding first focusing on the things you have complete control over, like your attitude and your nutrition; second, concentrating on concerns like pace targets; and lastly, outcomes, with the point being that finish times fall out of the first two buckets. She kept the goal of Boston in the back of her mind, knowing it would be a long road. The first year was a huge success and she made tremendous progress in her racing and results.

Sometime between year one and year two her thought process began to change. I could feel that her mental state had begun to switch to a more outcome-based thought process. As we were planning for year two, she began asking questions related to Boston qualification. She wanted to know which races gave her the best shot, and was willing to go to those events even if it meant undermining her long-term progress. I knew that she still needed to shave 10 to 15 minutes off her finish time to have a legitimate shot at Boston qualification. I spoke to her about this, but she decided that she still wanted to give it a go. As the season began, other stresses in her life become significant as she was finishing her PhD. She continued on the path of increasing training stress, with a likely reduced available stress budget due to school commitments. As we got closer to the first race of the year she began asking questions like "How much weight do

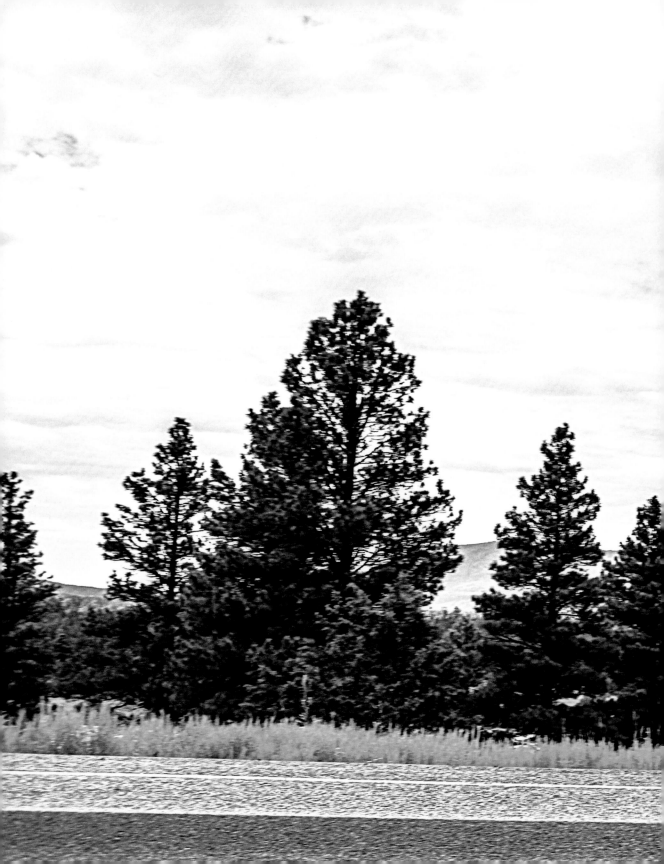

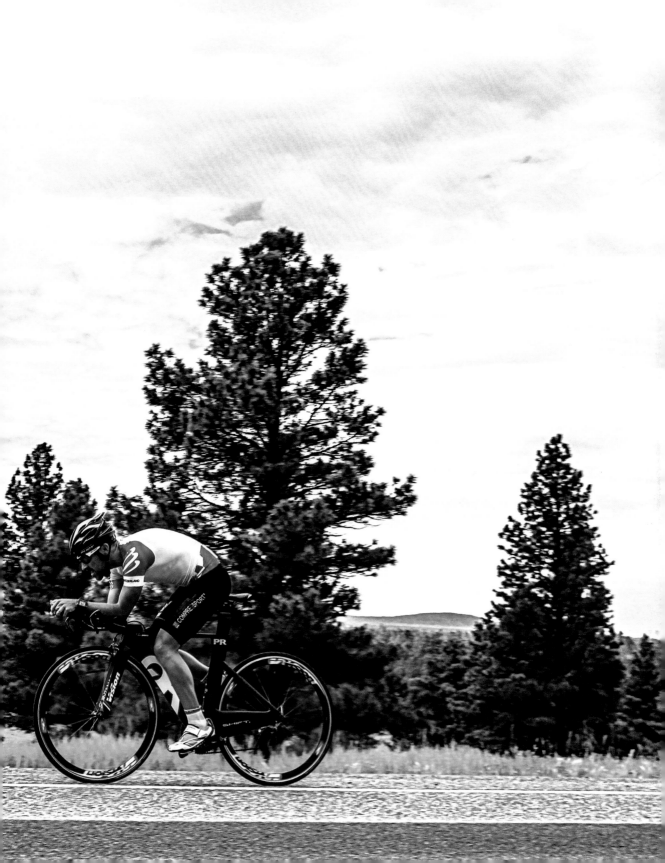

you think I can lose in the next six weeks?" and "How much faster would I go if I were X pounds lighter?" When checking her food intake menus I'd find that she was always undercutting planned protein, carbohydrate, and fat needs. She also began looking at the start rosters in great detail and frequently sent me lists of the athletes in her age group, including their previous results, and asked if she could beat them. Finally, as she began to taper for race day, she consistently overshot her training ranges and asked, "Can I do more race effort pickups? I feel I need those to race well next week." If her assigned heart rate range for a workout was 150 to 160 beats per minute (bpm), she'd always average 159 bpm, meaning that she had spent a good portion at a higher intensity than planned. So you can see that she was applying a tremendous amount of self-imposed pressure, in a situation where she really didn't have a good shot at her outcome-related goal. Because of the self-imposed pressures, she was making intensity and nutrition mistakes leading into race day. She had created a proverbial pressure cooker.

As race week approached, I knew she was in trouble and that too much tightening of her nutrition and adding physical stress during a period of planned rest had created a difficult mental state with expectations that couldn't be met. Race day came and went with a disappointing finish time. She was slower than the previous season, despite a great improvement in her training metrics. For a coach or athlete, this is a frustrating situation to be in and often leads to the athlete placing blame on the training program, with the claim that they simply didn't work hard enough. You can see that once this downward spiral begins, it can ultimately force the athlete from the sport. In Jane's case, that is exactly what happened. She finished out the season and then decided that marathon racing just wasn't for her.

I encourage age-group athletes to live a balanced lifestyle where health is achieved first, then focus on consistency in training and race results, and finally speed. Patience truly is a virtue. I see too many athletes taking the opposite approach by rushing outcome-focused goals, which can add the external pressures that lead to the endurance athlete triad—and many times the more serious female athlete triad, too. Athletes who focus on the process and the items they have 100% control over ultimately reduce their externally applied pressures and end up meeting their long-term goals.

STRESS AND GI HEALTH

The GI system plays the most significant role in the absorption of nutrients from the foods that we eat. Poor GI health results in the body's inability to get the macronutrients and micronutrients that it needs, sometimes to the point of considerable deficiencies. Perhaps even more obvious is the effect that GI health has on comfort. We have all experienced the discomforts associated with an unhealthy gut— be it pains associated with gas or worse, it ain't a good time. Another thing that a healthy gut enables you to do is apply and absorb training stress. It's hard to even get out there and exercise at all with the discomfort that comes from an unhappy GI system. Gas pains or the need to

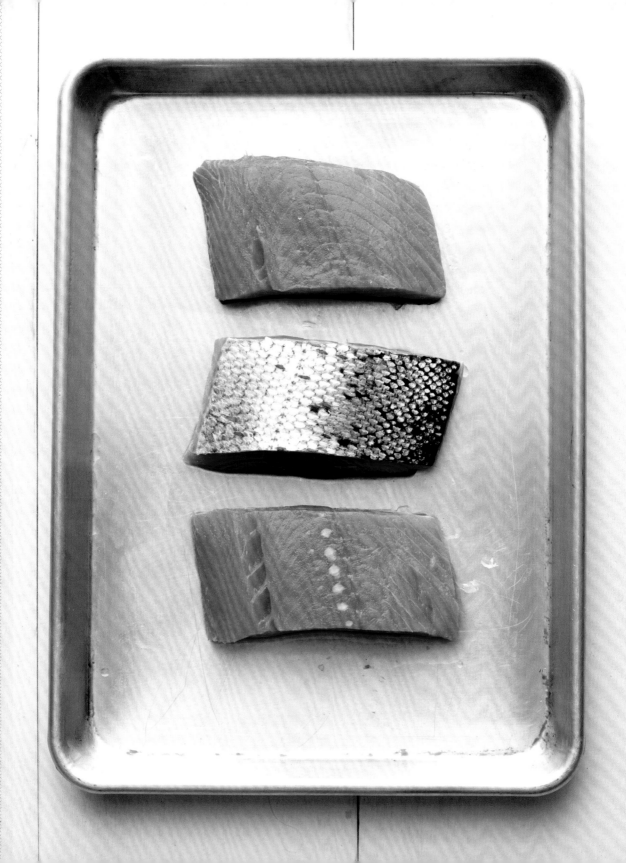

evacuate at inconvenient times, especially when brought on by the physical activity itself, are all telltale signs of a struggling GI tract. Training fuels can be a primary trigger of GI distress, as large amounts of sugar can provide a breeding ground for bad bacteria. A healthy gut is much more likely to be able to handle the fuels required for the sport. These fuels can be bothersome to a vulnerable GI system. So there are more than enough reasons for an endurance athlete to take a moment, especially during the time of year when training fuels are used heavily, to run a gut check and focus on turning the ship around, if needed.

Poor GI health typically manifests as bloating, food sensitivities, excessive fatigue, joint pain, headaches, weight gain, and an inability to handle training and racing fuels. While these symptoms may be present at any time, they will be further aggravated by any kind of stress, but especially the stress of intense workouts in preparation for an endurance race. Symptoms like bloating, joint pain, and headaches are pretty obvious when they show up. However, food sensitivities, fatigue, and weight gain are much more subtle signs of a problem. With so many demands constantly pulling us in different directions, it's hard to attribute feelings of fatigue to an irritated gut.

Poor GI health can develop very easily. You don't have to be sickly to experience an unhealthy gut. Improper nutrition, too much stress, or a bacterial imbalance can all cause issues. Too much gluten, even for a nonsensitive person, can also be an issue for many athletes. These contributory factors promote chronic inflammation of the GI system, making it nearly impossible to absorb key nutrients and minerals from foods, triggering an autoimmune-like response and leading to frequent sickness. If, in our training, consistency is king, poor GI health is in direct conflict with that goal. It takes a bite out of our long-term progress. It undermines our ability to adapt to increasing levels of stress, which is the key to getting faster. Add to this a diminished capacity to process important training and racing fuels, and we are faced with a double-edged sword slashing at us. Less fueling means less opportunity to apply training stress, as our bodies simply won't have the necessary fuels to drive forward. Inconsistent training, coupled with reduced training loads, by volume and/or intensity, make any kind of improvement quickly slip away. Considering that the goal is just the opposite—to increase sustainable training load and frequency—a healthy GI system is required.

Following the way of eating that's promoted in this book will help an unhealthy GI system. A diet of fish, lean meats, lean dairy, fruits, vegetables, nuts, seeds, and legumes is extremely nutrient dense and provides the body with the essential minerals needed for sustained health. Most of these foods are easy on the body, though you may need to make alterations based on your specific sensitivities. The following are a few foods and supplements that you can incorporate if you're struggling with tummy issues.

YOGURT

Lean dairy that contains active cultures, such as yogurt, can provide the body with good bacteria that promotes gut health. The active cultures *L. bulgaricus*, *S. thermophilus*, and *Bifidobacterium lactis* (aka *Bifidus regularis*) are commonly found in store-bought yogurts, and all create an environment that greatly eases digestion. Many enthusiasts believe that these active cultures boost immunity to infection, reduce cholesterol, and even serve as an anticarcinogen. Choose yogurts that are low in fat and have few added sugars, and look for a label that states that the active cultures are there, since not all yogurts have them.

STRESS REDUCTION

One of the most effective ways to improve GI health has very little to do with diet and everything to do with reducing stress. Chronic stress can have a tremendously negative impact on our gut health, going so far as to drastically change the way in which it functions. Stress may even increase the amount of poor bacteria in our gut, which deteriorates our digestive capabilities.

As driven athletes, we try to maintain our sport on top of the demands of family, work, friends, and myriad other things. And we're continually putting our body through significant physical stress, which demands a lot of sleep that we may not be getting. But something has to give. Take a close look at your patterns of living, talk with those who are closest to you, and find ways to make positive changes in order to decrease the overall stress in your life.

SUPPLEMENTATION

I discussed supplements in detail previously (see page 37), so here I'll mention those that have some relevance to GI health.

Fish Oils

Not only are fish oils important for heart health and their beneficial anti-inflammatory properties, but they can also help to reduce specific inflammation within the GI system. Also, fish oils are a valuable addition to enhance the delicate balance of gut bacteria.

Glutamine

When the training load gets heavy, glutamine can play a significant role in boosting the immune system, reducing GI inflammation, and balancing bacteria levels in the gut. A daily dose of 5 grams of glutamine is a perfect addition to your postworkout recovery drink. If you are specifically working on your GI health, you may want to dose as high as 10 to 15 grams daily for 8 to 12 weeks.

Probiotics

Often prescribed alongside antibiotics (which decimate good and bad bacteria alike), probiotics are little powerhouses that foster the development of good bacteria in our GI tract. If you feel as though you are struggling through a period of poor gut health, as evidenced in the preceding discussion, it may be worthwhile to begin using a probiotic to try and turn things around. A supplement such as Klean Athlete Probiotic is a great option. Look for a product, like this one, that provides 10 to 15 billion CFU per day. (CFU stands for *colony-forming unit* and is a measurement of the good bacteria in the product.) For day-to-day gut health, 2 to 4 CFU is enough.

OTHER INDICATORS OF FATIGUE

If you sense that you are run down, by either poor nutrition, too much training stress, or a combination thereof, then you should consider getting some blood work done. You may also want to get blood work before beginning training to be sure that you are in a position to properly absorb training stress. The table on the opposite page includes a list of blood markers that you can typically get from your general health care provider (the exception is the fatty acids, although these can be found online fairly inexpensively) and will help you determine if you are eating well and in a position to begin adding significant training stress.

To be clear, these markers are *not* used to determine health status or check for disease. They simply provide a look into your blood work as it relates to your performance as an endurance athlete. I've been using markers for many years, and they tend to cover the bases. I will say that in all the years I've been doing this, overtraining is way less common than under-resting.

RECIPES FOR PUTTING NUTRITION INTO PRACTICE

The following section of the book contains the recipes that I have relied on for years to support my own training and racing, and they are what I share with the athletes I work with. Shirley Fan, MS, RDN, helped pull the concepts together, developing and testing all of the dishes to ensure that they are the best they can be. Created to fit the characteristics and concepts discussed in this book, these recipes either contain only core foods or are core-ratio-friendly, except for those found in the Natural Workout Fueling section. I hope that these recipes are helpful tools for all athletes to achieve their peak health and performance—and that each one is enjoyed!

A NOTE ON REST

Rest and restorative techniques are the "secret" to making progress and creating big performances in your racing. What are restorative techniques? Anything an athlete does to create an environment in your body to recover and build the capacity to add more training stress: massage, hydration, sleep, and—the biggest one of all—nutrition! What we consume can help create a healthy system that allows bodies to heal, grow stronger, and handle more and more intense workouts. The athletes that can apply and absorb the most training stress make the most progress.

Restorative techniques are also rest days or weeks sprinkled throughout a training schedule. These "unload periods" are essential to allow athletes to apply bigger training loads when it counts most—the key training days. It's important for an athlete to have the courage to take rest days and weeks seriously.

BLOOD MARKERS FOR ASSESSING AN ATHLETE'S NUTRITION NEEDS

MARKER	BENCHMARK VALUE	PURPOSE
Hemoglobin	>13.5 g/dc	To assess O_2-carrying capacity
Ferritin (serum)	>50 ng/mL	To assess potential onset of iron anemia
Total iron-binding capacity	<375 mg/dc	To assess whether observed anemia could be due to disease
Cortisol*	<20 (7–8 a.m.) mcg/dc 7–28 mg/dc <17 (3–5 p.m.) mcg/dc 2–18 mg/dc	To assess chronic fatigue related to training load
Serum iron	>100 mcg/dc	To assess iron anemia
RBC magnesium	>4 mg/dc	To assess potential deficiency from electrolyte loss
25-hydroxy vitamin D	>35 ng/mL	To assess potential for stress fractures and limited performance
Calcium	>9 mg/dL	To assess potential for stress fractures
Transferrin saturation (percentage of open transferrin, a glycoprotein used to transport iron)	>20%	To assess iron anemia
Transferrin	<280 mg/dL	To assess iron anemia
MCV	<98 fL/RBC	To assess potential vitamin B_{12} anemia related to lack of red meat consumption
AA (arachidonic acid)	<9%	To assess intake of omega-6 fatty acids and quality of diet
EPA (eicosapentaenoic acid)	>4%	To assess intake of omega-3 fatty acids
AA/EPA	<4.0	To access cellular inflammation potential

* Cortisol that is too low is not beneficial. Typically when athletes begin to overtrain, cortisol increases. If it is pushed too far, it can drop severely. Be cautious in evaluating this marker.

REC

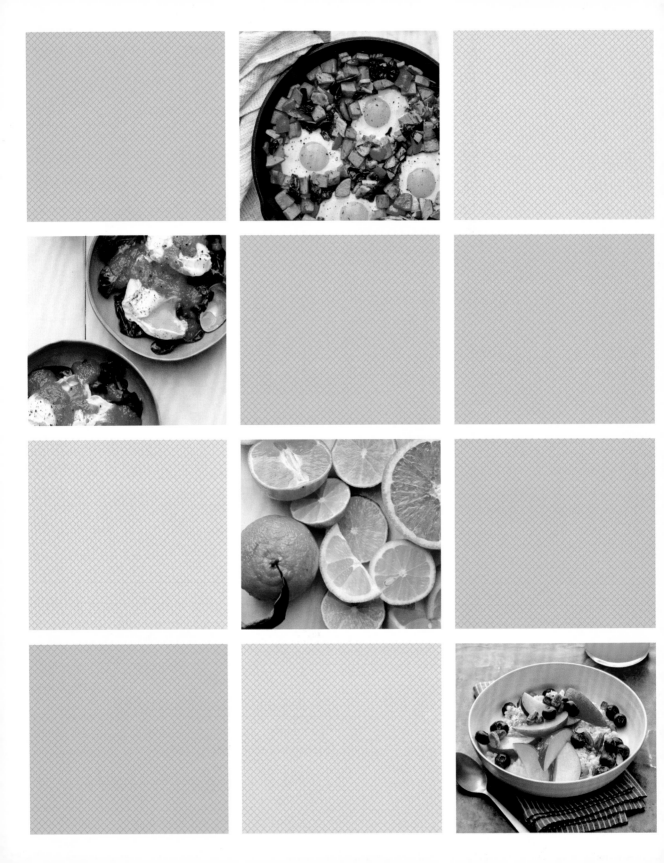

BREAKFAST

**PEACH AND BLUEBERRY
COTTAGE CHEESE BOWL**

99

**COCONUT CHIA SEED
PUDDING**

100

**HIGH-PROTEIN
PANCAKES**

102

**SPICED QUINOA
WITH APPLES AND
WALNUTS**

103

**POACHED EGGS WITH
RED PEPPER SAUCE AND
GARLICKY SPINACH**

105

**HARD-BOILED EGGS
WITH HERB SALT**

106

**MUSHROOM AND
HERB FRITTATA**

107

**SWEET POTATO HASH
WITH EGGS**

108

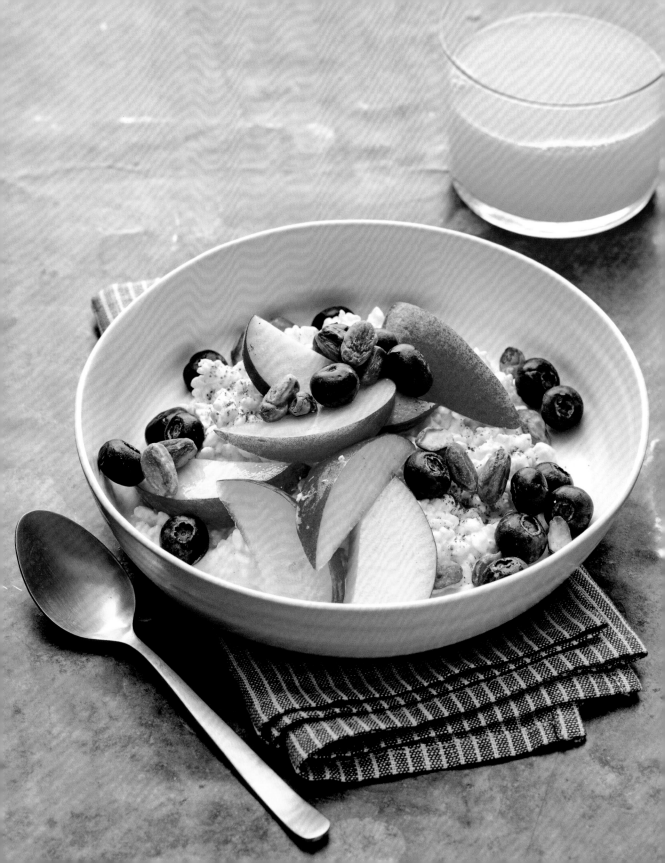

PEACH AND BLUEBERRY
COTTAGE CHEESE BOWL

SERVES 2

PER SERVING

CALORIES: 204.2
FAT: 4.3 g
SODIUM: 587.2 mg
CARBOHYDRATE: 20.2 g
FIBER: 2.7 g
SUGARS: 13.4 g
PROTEIN: 24.7 g

When peaches are in season, they are incredibly sweet and just plain delicious. In this dish, juicy slices of fresh peaches and plump blueberries top a lightly spiced cottage cheese. With a sprinkling of pistachios, this is a satisfying protein-packed and antioxidant-rich meal.

When fruits and vegetables are out of season, opt for frozen. Unlike canned produce, which can lose a lot of nutrients through processing, frozen fruits and vegetables tend to be picked and frozen at their peak.

1½ cups low-fat cottage cheese
Pinch of ground cinnamon
Pinch of ground nutmeg
1 medium ripe peach, pitted, peeled, and sliced, or 1 cup frozen unsweetened peach slices, thawed
½ cup fresh blueberries or frozen blueberries, thawed
2 tablespoons toasted pistachios (see Tip)

IN A MEDIUM BOWL, combine the cottage cheese, cinnamon, and nutmeg. Evenly divide the cottage cheese between two serving bowls. Top with sliced peaches, blueberries, and pistachios. Serve.

TIP: To toast nuts, spread them in a single layer on a baking sheet and place in a 350°F. oven. Roast for 5 minutes, then stir. Check the nuts every 2 to 3 minutes. They should smell nutty, look golden, and begin making crackling sounds when done. Alternatively, you can toast small amounts of nuts on the stovetop. Place the nuts in a dry skillet set over medium heat and toast, stirring constantly, until nutty and golden brown, about 5 minutes.

PER SERVING

CALORIES: 236.5
FAT: 8.6 g
SODIUM: 51.8 mg
CARBOHYDRATE: 41.6 g
FIBER: 10 g
SUGARS: 26.1 g
PROTEIN: 5.5 g

COCONUT CHIA SEED PUDDING

SERVES 6

½ cup chia seeds
2 to 2¼ cups unsweetened vanilla coconut milk (see Tip)
2 medium bananas
6 to 8 medjool dates, chopped
¼ cup toasted unsweetened coconut flakes

Start the day off right with a mix of protein and fiber from this tropical breakfast pudding that is similar to tapioca. It's great after a workout, thanks to the potassium-rich banana and dates, which can help replenish lost electrolytes and reenergize the body. Chia seeds contain numerous healthy nutrients as well, including omega-3 fatty acids that help reduce cellular inflammation, and great calcium content to support bone health.

IN A LARGE BOWL OR MASON JAR, combine the chia seeds and coconut milk. Whisk or shake together until well incorporated. Cover and refrigerate overnight.

SPOON THE PUDDING into 6 serving dishes and divide the bananas, dates, and coconut flakes over the top of each.

TIP: If the pudding is too thick or thin for your taste, adjust the liquid. I also like to top it off with extra coconut milk before serving, so I can mix in a little myself once I'm ready to eat!

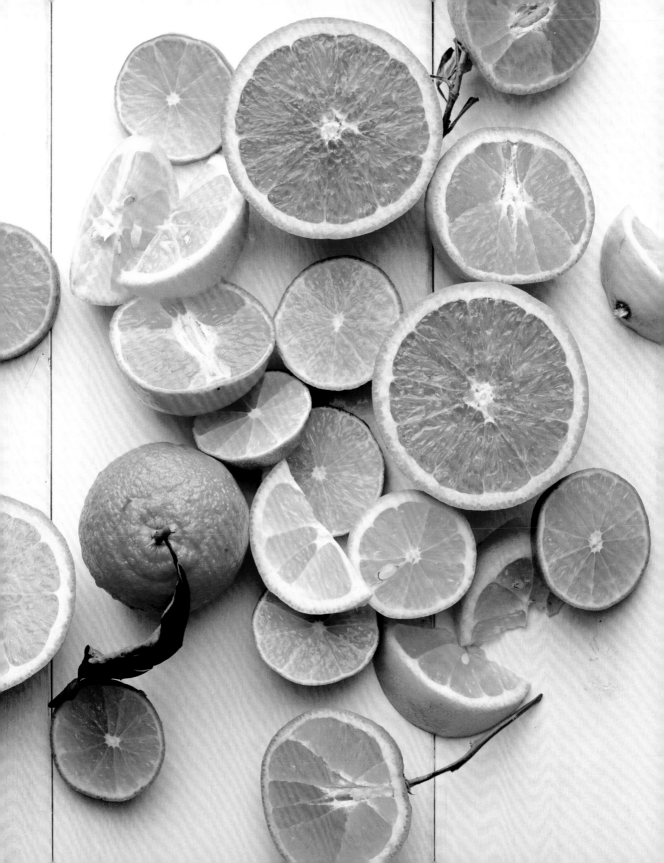

HIGH-PROTEIN
PANCAKES

MAKES SIX 5-INCH PANCAKES: SERVES 2

3 large eggs (see Tip)
2 large egg whites
1 teaspoon vanilla
   extract
½ cup fat-free
   cottage cheese
1 cup oat flour
Nonstick cooking
   spray

These pancakes are extremely low in their glycemic load because of the significant protein content from cottage cheese and egg whites. Although they are not a true core food (see page 18), they are low enough on the glycemic load scale to enjoy as if they are. This is a great recipe for those weekend mornings that may be a recovery day, or even those Monday mornings after a big weekend of training when you want a bit more protein for muscle protein synthesis. I like to serve them with a sprinkle of blueberries and agave nectar instead of syrup.

IN A MEDIUM BOWL, whisk together the eggs, egg whites, and vanilla. Whisk in the cottage cheese. Using a rubber spatula, gently stir in the oat flour. (Alternatively, the ingredients can be combined in a blender for a smoother pancake.)

SPRAY A LARGE NONSTICK SKILLET with cooking spray and set it over medium heat. Using a ¼-cup measure, scoop a heaping amount of the batter into the pan. Tilt the pan slightly to even out the batter. Cook until the pancake begins to bubble, the edges look dry, and the bottom is lightly browned, about 3 minutes. Flip, and cook for 1 more minute. Transfer to a plate and repeat with the remaining batter.

TIP: Long vilified for high cholesterol content, eggs are now touted as one of the most convenient and cheapest sources of quality protein. One large egg contains 6 grams of protein, which can keep us satiated for a long time and help with muscle building and repair. I recommend choosing fortified eggs when possible, as they include more omega-3s than other varieties.

SPICED QUINOA
WITH APPLES AND WALNUTS

SERVES 4

PER SERVING

CALORIES: 335.7
FAT: 9.7 g
SODIUM: 131.4 mg
CARBOHYDRATE: 53.6 g
FIBER: 5.2 g
SUGARS: 22.5 g
PROTEIN: 11.4 g

1 cup quinoa
2 cups 1% milk
¾ teaspoon ground cinnamon
⅛ teaspoon coarse salt
½ tablespoon light butter (see Tip)
2 medium apples, cored and thinly sliced
1 teaspoon fresh lemon juice
¼ cup toasted chopped walnuts (see Tip, page 99)
4 teaspoons honey

If you're not a fan of eggs, starting a nonworkout day with a protein-packed breakfast can be a challenge. Recently I discovered that you can use quinoa to make an oatmeal-like porridge. All you need to do is cook it with more liquid so that it takes on the right consistency. In this recipe, I add a few things to amp up the flavor, but you should experiment with ingredients you like. If you enjoy planning your breakfast ahead, the quinoa can be made 1 to 2 days before, and rewarmed over low heat. (Thin it down with more water or milk if it's too thick.)

RINSE THE QUINOA under running water until the water is clear. Transfer the quinoa to a medium pot. Add 2 cups water, the milk, ½ teaspoon of the cinnamon, and the salt. Bring to a boil over medium heat, reduce the heat to low, and simmer until the quinoa is tender, 20 to 25 minutes. Meanwhile, in a large nonstick skillet or sauté pan set over medium heat, melt the butter. Add the apples, lemon juice, and the remaining ¼ teaspoon cinnamon. Cook the apples until tender, 5 to 7 minutes.

TO SERVE, divide the quinoa among four serving bowls. Place the apples and walnuts over the top, and drizzle with honey.

TIP: In place of butter in many recipes, I like to use a product I call *light butter*. Found in most grocery stores, light butter, like Smart Balance, is made with oils that contain healthy omega-3 fatty acids and a much lower content of saturated fat.

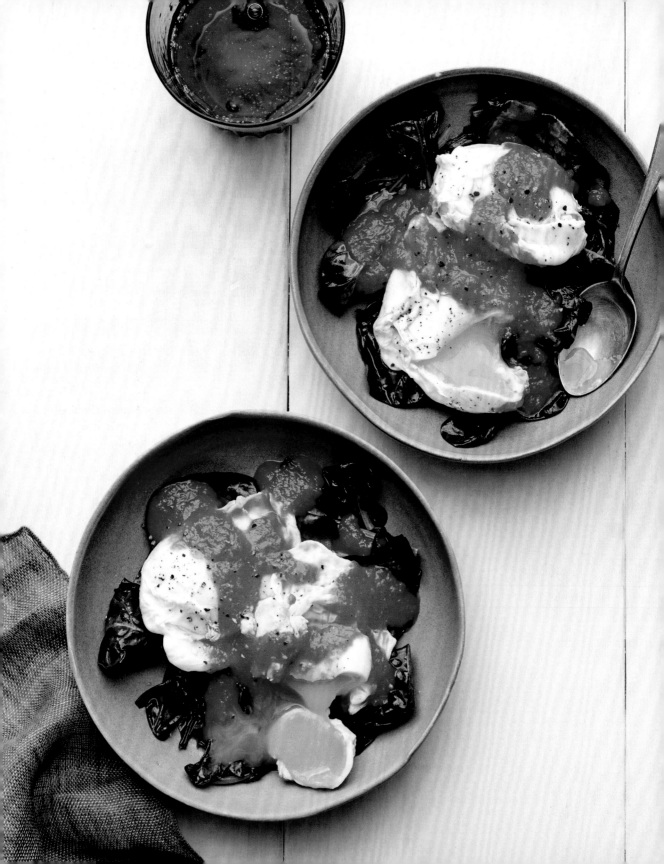

POACHED EGGS
WITH RED PEPPER SAUCE AND GARLICKY SPINACH

SERVES 2

PER SERVING

CALORIES: 196.8
FAT: 14.5 g
SODIUM: 354.4 mg
CARBOHYDRATE: 8.3 g
FIBER: 2.4 g
SUGARS: 3.1 g
PROTEIN: 10.3 g

Of the ways to prepare eggs, poaching can be either one of the easiest or trickiest methods. It involves cooking eggs in simmering liquid until the whites are firm and the yolks are runny. I've had my share of mishaps in making poached eggs, but the best part is that eggs are fairly inexpensive and you can always try again (or just eat your mistakes!).

¾ cup jarred roasted red pepper, drained (about 4 ounces)
3 garlic cloves
2 tablespoons extra-virgin olive oil
1 tablespoon red wine vinegar
1 tablespoon distilled white vinegar
4 large eggs
1 (5-ounce) package of fresh baby spinach

IN THE BOWL OF A FOOD PROCESSOR, combine the roasted red pepper, 1 of the garlic cloves, 1 tablespoon of the oil, and the red wine vinegar. Process until smooth.

FILL A DEEP 12-INCH SAUTÉ PAN with enough water to come 1 inch up the sides of the pan. Set the pan over medium heat and bring the water to a simmer. Stir in the white vinegar.

ONE AT A TIME, crack each egg into a small cup or ramekin, then gently drop each egg into the simmering water, making sure they aren't too close to one another. Turn off the heat and let cook until the whites are cooked and the yolks are soft and runny, 5 minutes. Using a slotted spoon, transfer the eggs to a plate; keep warm.

POUR THE WATER out of the pan, and set the pan over medium-high heat. Add the remaining 1 tablespoon oil. Chop the remaining 2 garlic cloves and cook in the oil until fragrant, 30 seconds. Add the spinach and cook until just wilted, 2 to 3 minutes. Divide the spinach between two serving plates. Top with two poached eggs, spoon the sauce on top, and serve.

HARD-BOILED EGGS
WITH HERB SALT

SERVES 6

¼ cup kosher salt
¼ cup packed fresh herbs, such as parsley, tarragon, basil, or cilantro
½ teaspoon lemon or lime zest
12 large eggs

For most athletes, nonworkout mornings are typically recovery days, which follow hard training days. Starting off one of those nonworkout mornings with a couple of hard-boiled eggs is a great way to get good-quality protein into your body to facilitate muscle protein synthesis and recovery! While one can't argue against salt and pepper seasoning, we discovered an interesting and flavorful way to jazz up eggs: homemade herb salt. Simply blend salt and fresh herbs with ingredients like citrus zest to create a flavorful salt. You can easily make a large batch of herb salt to save for other dishes or to give to friends and family (see Tip).

PREHEAT THE OVEN to 200°F.

IN THE BOWL OF A MINI FOOD PROCESSOR or blender, combine the salt, herbs, and zest. Process until the leaves are finely chopped and incorporated into the salt. Scatter the salt onto a baking sheet. Bake until dry, 10 minutes. (You can also let the salt dry at room temperature for 1 hour.)

GENTLY PLACE THE EGGS in a large saucepan. Add enough water to cover by 1 inch. Cover the pan and bring to a rolling boil. Turn off the heat and let the eggs sit in the water, with the pan covered, until cooked through, 11 minutes.

COOL THE EGGS under cool running water and remove the shells. Slice the eggs in half and sprinkle a pinch of the herb salt (1/16 teaspoon) over each egg.

TIP: Store the remaining salt in an airtight container. It will keep for 6 months.

MUSHROOM AND HERB FRITTATA

SERVES 8

I love this easy-to-make dish because it's so flavorful and versatile. It can be enjoyed on its own for breakfast or served with a green salad for lunch. Feel free to use other herbs such as tarragon or basil, substitute other types of mushrooms and cheese, or add veggies like spinach, broccoli, or kale.

PREHEAT THE BROILER. Set the rack to the top.

IN A 12-INCH NONSTICK, OVENPROOF SKILLET set over medium-high heat, heat 1 tablespoon of the oil. Add the mushrooms and garlic, and cook until soft, about 5 minutes. Transfer to a small bowl, and let cool for 10 minutes.

IN A MEDIUM BOWL, beat the eggs and egg whites with a fork. Stir in the mushrooms and garlic, Parmesan, salt, and pepper.

SET THE SAME PAN over medium heat, and add the remaining 1 tablespoon oil. Pour the egg mixture into the pan, and cook, stirring with a heatproof rubber spatula. Add the herbs and continue to cook for about 5 minutes, or until the eggs begin to set on the bottom. Run the spatula underneath the eggs to make sure they aren't sticking to the pan.

TRANSFER THE PAN to the broiler and broil until the frittata is browned on top, about 2 minutes. Slide the frittata onto a cutting board, cut into 8 wedges, and serve.

TIP: I always recommend that athletes use two egg whites for every whole egg, because it helps them get the egg's quality protein and the yolk's nutrient density, but without overdoing the saturated fat found in the yolk.

PER SERVING

CALORIES: 90.8
FAT: 6.4 g
SODIUM: 247.3 mg
CARBOHYDRATE: 1.5 g
FIBER: 0.3 g
SUGARS: 0.8 g
PROTEIN: 7.3 g

2 tablespoons extra-virgin olive oil
8 ounces sliced crimini mushrooms
1 garlic clove, chopped
3 large eggs
6 large egg whites (see Tip)
¼ cup grated Parmesan cheese
½ teaspoon coarse salt
¼ teaspoon freshly ground black pepper
1 tablespoon chopped fresh flat-leaf parsley
1 tablespoon chopped chives

SWEET POTATO HASH
WITH EGGS

SERVES 2

1 tablespoon olive oil
½ small yellow onion, chopped
3 slices Canadian bacon (see Tip), chopped (about 2 ounces)
½ teaspoon dried thyme
1 large sweet potato, peeled and cut into ½-inch cubes (about 12 ounces)
½ medium red bell pepper, cored, seeded, and chopped
¼ teaspoon plus ⅛ teaspoon coarse salt
¼ teaspoon plus ⅛ teaspoon freshly ground black pepper
2 cups packed baby spinach
4 large eggs

Although Canadian bacon contains the word *bacon*, it's actually more like thick ham. In fact, Canadian bacon, or *back bacon*, comes from the middle back side of the animal, making it much leaner than bacon, which is cut from the side of the pig. But it still has a great smoky flavor and works really well in this filling breakfast hash.

IN A LARGE NONSTICK SAUTÉ PAN or seasoned cast-iron pan over medium-high heat, heat the oil. When the oil begins to shimmer, add the onion and cook until soft, about 5 minutes. Add the bacon and thyme, and cook for 1 to 2 more minutes. Add the sweet potato and bell pepper, and season with ¼ teaspoon each of the salt and pepper. Reduce the heat to medium, cover the pan, and cook, stirring occasionally, until the potatoes are tender and starting to brown, 10 to 15 minutes. Fold in the spinach and cook until it begins to wilt, about 2 minutes. Crack each egg into the four corners of the pan. Cover and cook for 5 minutes, or until desired doneness. Season each egg with the ⅛ teaspoon salt and ⅛ teaspoon pepper.

TO SERVE, divide the eggs and hash between two serving plates.

TIP: I sometimes keep store-bought precooked Canadian bacon patties in the fridge to have as a quick cold snack on their own, or with core-ratio-friendly crackers and low-fat cheese.

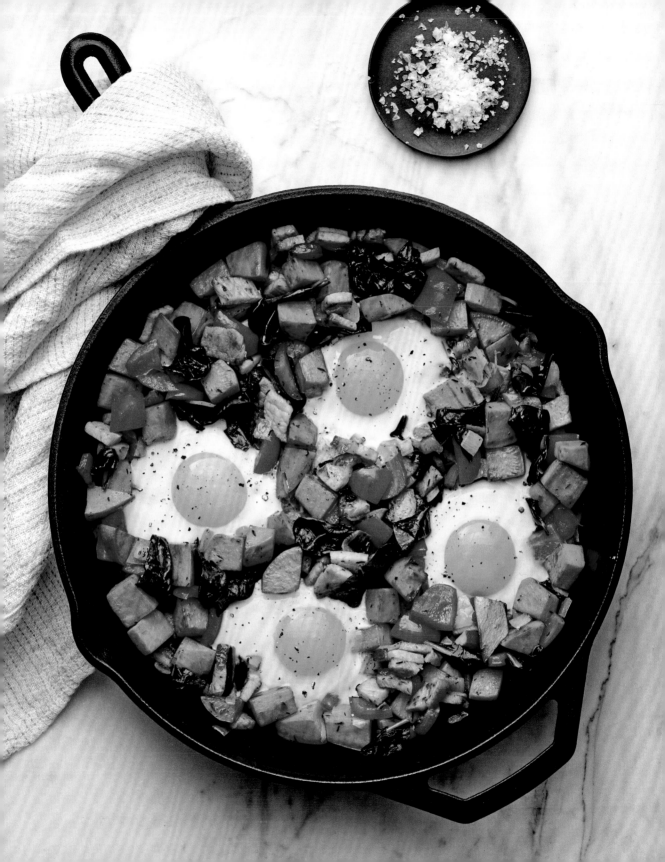

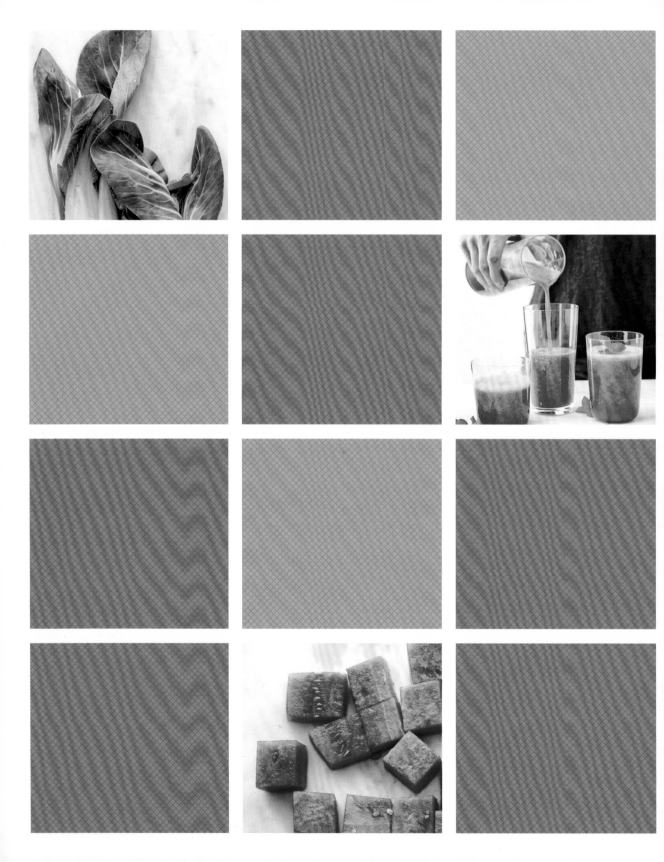

JUICES & SMOOTHIES

PER SERVING

CALORIES: 249.6
FAT: 2.2 g
SODIUM: 120 mg
CARBOHYDRATE: 49.8 g
FIBER: 3.8 g
SUGARS: 13.8 g
PROTEIN: 11 g

TRIPLE GREEN JUICE

MAKES ONE 16-OUNCE DRINK

½ medium cucumber, chopped (about 6 ounces)
1 medium apple, chopped
4 large stalks kale
2 cups packed baby spinach (about 2 ounces)
1-inch piece fresh ginger, chopped

I have been juicing for years, and as odd as it may sound, it can be a therapeutic break in a hectic day. For athletes, the benefits of juicing run pretty deep. Juicing fruits and vegetables provides a huge dose of phytonutrients (plant chemicals) in a concentrated, easily absorbed form. This quality alone makes juicing whole, fresh, and raw fruits and vegetables one of the most powerful vehicles for achieving optimal health. Some other benefits include increased hydration, quick and easy absorption of nutrients, and delivery of helpful enzymes and chlorophyll (found exclusively in plants). For athletes who have a lot on their plates, and who are working to adapt nutritious eating habits, I put juicing pretty low on the priority list. However, for athletes who eat well regularly, I recommend juicing as a great way to supplement!

FEED THE CUCUMBER THROUGH A JUICER (see Tip), followed by the apple, kale, spinach, and ginger. Stir to combine. Drink within 1 day.

TIP: Owning a juicer isn't necessary to create your own juices at home. In fact, all you need is a blender. Simply puree all the ingredients together in a blender, and then strain the pulp through a fine-mesh sieve or nut milk bag (find either online or at a kitchen supply store).

BLUEBERRY
PROTEIN SMOOTHIE

MAKES ONE 24-OUNCE SMOOTHIE

PER SERVING

CALORIES: 295.6
FAT: 3.3 g
SODIUM: 89 mg
CARBOHYDRATE: 50.8 g
FIBER: 4.9 g
SUGARS: 15.1 g
PROTEIN: 18.8 g

Blueberries are one of the most nutrient-dense sources of carbohydrates known to humankind, and they're packed with antioxidants. As an endurance athlete, you create plenty of free radicals with the activities you do, so antioxidants that can help prevent cell damage from these free radicals are a welcomed addition. This simple protein-fruit smoothie is an easy way to get a solid dose.

1 cup no-sugar-added apple or grape juice
1 level scoop vanilla whey protein powder
1 cup frozen blueberries (see Tip)

IN A BLENDER, combine the juice, protein powder, and blueberries. Blend for 30 seconds or until smooth and frothy.

TIP: Have an abundance of fresh blueberries? Why not freeze them? Wash them, and then arrange in a single layer on a sheet pan. Freeze for 1 to 2 hours, then transfer to a resealable plastic bag.

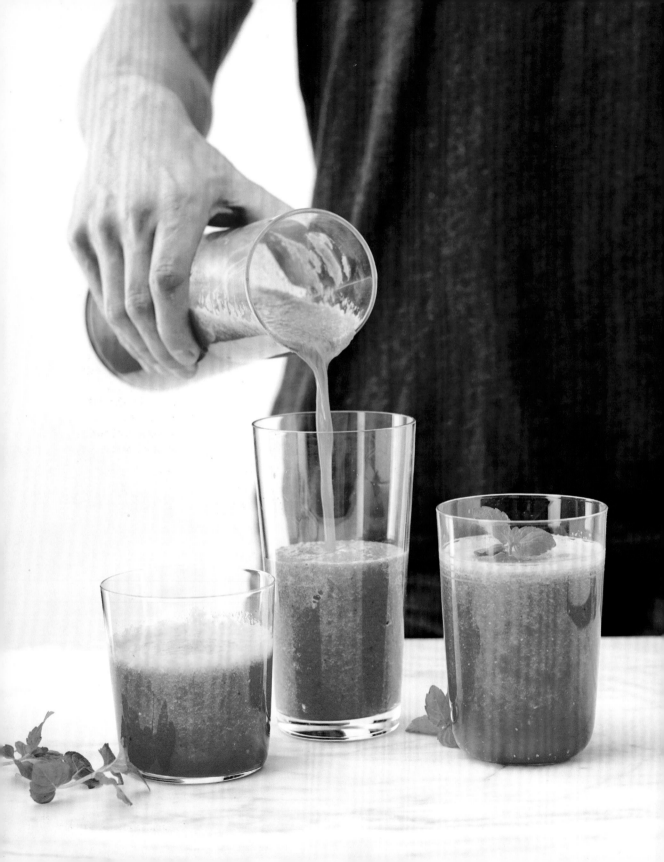

WATERMELON, LIME, AND MINT JUICE

MAKES TWO 8-OUNCE DRINKS; SERVES 2

A summertime mainstay, watermelon is immensely refreshing. For the athlete, watermelon is great for hydration in the summer, as it's largely (about 92%) made of water. Research also suggests that it may help soothe sore muscles, thanks to an amino acid called L-citrulline that helps relax blood vessels and improve circulation. Better yet, it provides boosts of vitamin C, beta-carotene, and lycopene, an antioxidant that may help fight chronic disease. Try this juice when you're looking for a postworkout refresher. I have a friend with a fairly high sweat rate who would honestly consume half a watermelon every day in the summer when in heavy training as a way to stay hydrated!

2½ cups cubed seedless watermelon (about 1 pound)
1 tablespoon fresh lime juice
5 to 8 fresh mint leaves
2 fresh mint sprigs, for garnish

IN A BLENDER, combine the watermelon, lime juice, and mint leaves and blend until smooth and frothy. Serve in small tumblers and garnish with a mint sprig.

PER SERVING

CALORIES: 371.3
FAT: 4.8 g
SODIUM: 189.8 mg
CARBOHYDRATE: 59.5 g
FIBER: 3.6 g
SUGARS: 46.4 g
PROTEIN: 27.5 g

BANANA-HONEY
PROTEIN SMOOTHIE

MAKES ONE 20-OUNCE SMOOTHIE

1 cup unsweetened 1% milk

1 level scoop vanilla whey protein powder, such as Designer Whey

1 frozen medium ripe banana (see Tip)

1 tablespoon honey or agave nectar (optional)

This protein-packed smoothie can be served for breakfast on nonworkout mornings or between meals. The protein powder adds 18 grams of protein to help facilitate muscle protein synthesis, keep blood sugar stable, and keep you satiated for hours. Many of the athletes I have worked with over the years love an easy, hearty smoothie such as this one that they can turn to for a quick snack almost any time between workouts!

IN A BLENDER, combine the milk, protein powder, banana, and honey (if using). Blend for 30 seconds or until smooth and frothy.

TIP: Mostly known for their potassium and anticramping effects, bananas are also a source of fiber, vitamins B_6 and C, magnesium, and folate. Because of their natural sweetness, I like to keep a stash of peeled bananas in my freezer for smoothies or baked goods. Simply remove the peel from ripe bananas and keep them in a resealable plastic bag in the freezer. Almost all smoothies turn out better when you use frozen fruit instead of ice!

COCOA, ALMOND, AND
DATE SMOOTHIE

MAKES ONE 10-OUNCE SMOOTHIE

PER SERVING

CALORIES: 159.6
FAT: 2.9 g
SODIUM: 181.3 mg
CARBOHYDRATE: 36.4 g
FIBER: 5.2 g
SUGARS: 28.2 g
PROTEIN: 2.4 g

Dates are incredibly sweet and have a sticky, chewy texture, making them ideal for baked goods, chutneys, granola, salads, pilafs, and spreads. Because I prefer natural sources of sugar that come with some nutrient density, I use them to sweeten this chocolate-y smoothie. Soaking the dates ahead of time softens their chewy skin and helps make the drink smoother.

¼ cup packed pitted dates (see Tip)
1 cup unsweetened almond milk
1 teaspoon unsweetened cocoa powder
Ice cubes (optional)

PUT THE DATES AND ALMOND MILK in a small bowl and let soak until the dates are soft, about 15 minutes.

TRANSFER THE DATES AND ALMOND MILK to a blender and add the cocoa powder. Blend until smooth and frothy. Blend in a few ice cubes (if using) for an icy cold drink.

TIP: A source of dietary fiber, B vitamins, magnesium, and potassium, dates also contain easy-to-digest carbohydrates. Have them before a workout for a quick energy boost in place of an energy gel. They can even be used during exercise in moderation as a replacement for energy gels and bars.

NATURAL WORKOUT FUELING

ALTHOUGH I RECOMMEND FUELING WORKOUTS and races with performance products that contain adequate sodium, fluid, and carbohydrates (while being void of fat and fiber), some athletes prefer to fuel their workouts (considerably in advance of race day) with natural foods. The recipes in this section can be used for this purpose. Also, dates or flattened bananas can be consumed instead of sports bars or gels during workouts to fulfill any additional carbohydrate needs.

PUMPKIN-OAT
QUICK BREAD

MAKES 2 LOAVES: SERVES 16

Try eating this quick bread before a workout or even during a bike or swim workout to get a good mix of carbohydrates, protein, and fat. The applesauce and canned pumpkin keep it low in fat so that it can be quickly digested, which also keeps the focus on carbohydrates to fuel your workout! This is a great replacement for a typical sports energy bar.

PREHEAT THE OVEN to 325°F. Grease two 8½ × 4½-inch loaf pans with cooking spray or line them with parchment paper.

IN A MEDIUM BOWL, combine the flour, oats, protein powder, baking soda, cinnamon, and nutmeg. Set aside.

IN A LARGE BOWL, whisk together the eggs, honey, pumpkin, and applesauce. Gradually add the dry ingredients to the wet, and mix until just combined. Evenly divide the batter between the two prepared pans.

BAKE UNTIL GOLDEN and a toothpick inserted into the center of the bread comes out clean, 40 to 45 minutes. Let cool for 10 minutes before transferring the loaves to a wire rack. Let cool completely before cutting each loaf into 8 slices.

TIP: Honey can turn into a sweet and sticky mess when you are trying to remove it from measuring cups. An easy trick is to spray the inside of a measuring cup with cooking spray before pouring the honey. The oil will help the honey slide right out.

Nonstick cooking spray
1⅓ cups whole-wheat flour
½ cup quick-cooking oats
3 level scoops vanilla whey protein powder
1 teaspoon baking soda
1 teaspoon ground cinnamon
½ teaspoon ground nutmeg
2 large eggs
1 cup honey (see Tip)
1 cup canned pumpkin puree
½ cup unsweetened applesauce

PER SERVING

CALORIES: 136.7
FAT: 0.8 g
SODIUM: 102.2 mg
CARBOHYDRATE: 29 g
FIBER: 2.3 g
SUGARS: 19.1 g
PROTEIN: 5.8 g

HONEY-WALNUT
BANANA BREAD

MAKES 2 LOAVES: SERVES 16

Nonstick cooking spray
2 cups whole-wheat
   flour
3 level scoops vanilla
   whey protein
   powder (see Tip)
2 teaspoons baking
   powder
1 teaspoon ground
   cinnamon
¾ teaspoon baking
   soda
¾ teaspoon salt
½ teaspoon cream of
   tartar
2 large eggs
2 egg whites
⅓ cup skim milk
1 cup honey
3 tablespoons
   canola oil
3 tablespoons
   unsweetened
   applesauce
1½ cups mashed ripe
   bananas (about
   3 medium)
½ cup chopped walnuts

This quick bread is a great alternative to energy or granola bars, as whole-wheat flour for healthy carbs, whey powder for protein, and mashed bananas for sweetness and potassium (so many of the typical workout fuels are low on potassium, so it never hurts to load up before your workout). You can freeze one of the loaves, so you'll always have a healthy snack on hand.

PREHEAT THE OVEN to 325°F. Lightly grease two 8½ × 4½-inch loaf pans with cooking spray or line them with parchment paper.

IN A MEDIUM BOWL, combine the flour, protein powder, baking powder, cinnamon, baking soda, salt, and cream of tartar. Set aside.

IN A LARGE BOWL, whisk together the eggs, egg whites, milk, honey, oil, and applesauce. Gradually add the dry ingredients to the wet, and mix until just combined. Fold in the bananas and walnuts. Evenly divide the batter between the two prepared pans.

BAKE UNTIL GOLDEN and a toothpick inserted into the center of the bread comes out clean, about 45 minutes. Let cool 10 minutes before transferring the loaves to a wire rack. Let cool completely before cutting each loaf into 8 slices.

PER SERVING

CALORIES: 201.6
FAT: 5.7 g
SODIUM: 247 mg
CARBOHYDRATE: 35.2 g
FIBER: 2.8 g
SUGARS: 21 g
PROTEIN: 6 g

TIP: Whey is a by-product of cheese or yogurt making; it is the liquid that is left behind after the milk has been curdled and strained. Whey contains protein, minerals, vitamins, and sometimes lactose, which help with muscle building and repair. Whey protein powder is a convenient and concentrated form of whey; you can find it in vitamin shops and some supermarkets.

GRAPE JUICE
SPORTS DRINK

MAKES ONE 24-OUNCE DRINK

This super simple homemade sports drink requires almost no prep time at all. Grape juice is fairly high on the glycemic scale, so it's okay to drink during a workout or immediately postworkout only. With the addition of salt to increase the sodium content, it's a simple alternative to store-bought versions of the best sports drink mixes. Note that most watered-down fruit juices with added sodium can be used. Just target 40 to 50 grams of carbohydrate per 24 ounces, and add 500 to 600 milligrams of sodium.

1⅔ cups cold water
1⅓ cups cold no-sugar-added grape juice
⅛ teaspoon table salt (see Tip)

PER SERVING

CALORIES: 202
FAT: 0 g
SODIUM: 592 mg
CARBOHYDRATE: 49 g
FIBER: 0 g
SUGARS: 48 g
PROTEIN: 1 g

IN A SPORTS BOTTLE, combine the water, juice, and salt. Shake well.

TIP: For added trace minerals, replace the table salt with sea salt, such as BASE Performance brand Electrolyte Salt.

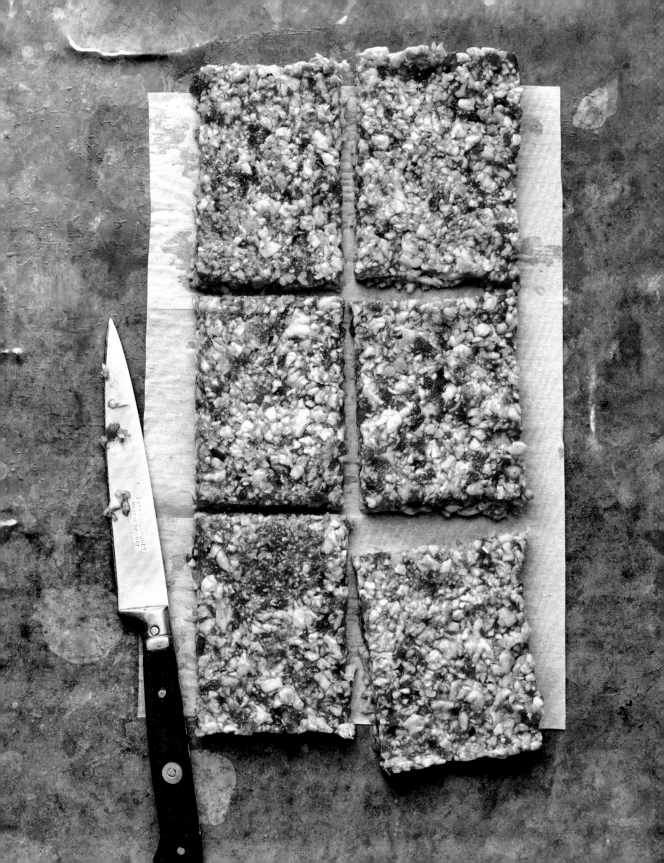

APPLE, CINNAMON, AND
DATE BARS

MAKES 6 BARS

Chewy, nutty, and fruity, these energy-dense bars are great for fueling a workout. Although some athletes with an iron gut may be able to handle these while running, they are likely best for cycling. They are naturally sweet, thanks to dates and apples, and have a hit of satisfying cashews. Make them ahead of time, and package them up individually in resealable plastic bags or waxed or parchment paper for easy portability.

Nonstick cooking spray
4 ounces pitted dates
3 ounces dried apples (see Tip)
½ teaspoon plus ⅛ teaspoon coarse salt
¼ teaspoon ground cinnamon
1¼ ounces raw or roasted unsalted cashews

LINE AN 8½ × 4½-INCH LOAF PAN with waxed or parchment paper, and lightly grease with cooking spray.

PUT THE DATES in a small bowl. Cover with warm water and soak for 15 to 30 minutes. Drain.

IN A FOOD PROCESSOR, combine the dates, apples, salt, and cinnamon. Process until the fruit begins to blend and stick together. Add the cashews and process again until the nuts break into smaller pieces. Transfer the mixture to the prepared pan and spread into an even layer. Refrigerate for at least 1 hour to set. Cut into 6 bars.

PER SERVING

CALORIES: 120
FAT: 2.5 g
SODIUM: 135 mg
CARBOHYDRATE: 25 g
FIBER: 3 g
SUGARS: 20 g
PROTEIN: 2 g

TIP: Have a surplus of apples? You can make your own dried apples at home by cutting peeled or unpeeled apples into ¼-inch slices and baking in a single layer in a 225°F. oven until dry and flexible, about 1½ hours, turning halfway through.

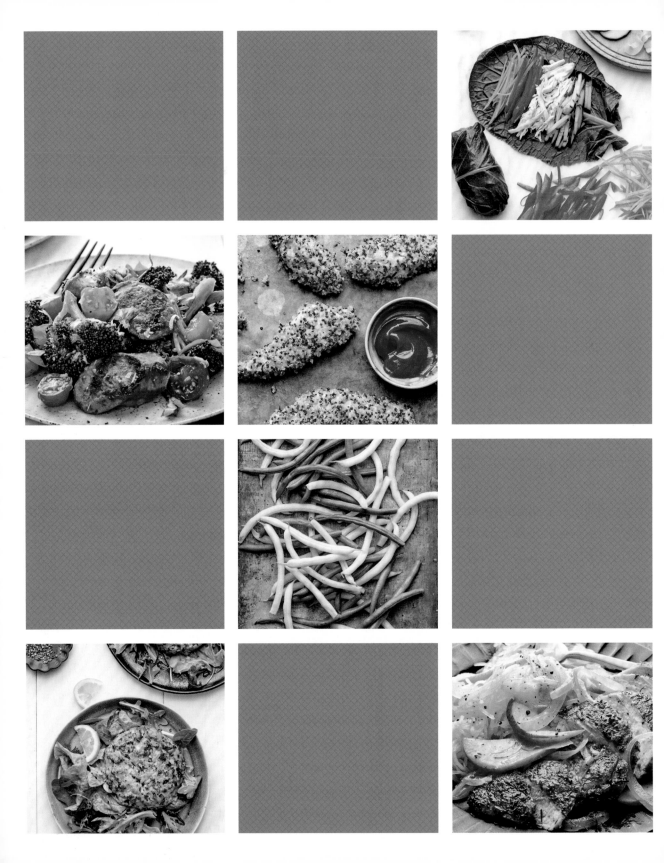

LUNCH

QUINOA
WITH ORANGE, CRANBERRIES, AND GOAT CHEESE

SERVES 4

1½ cups quinoa (see Tip)
1 medium orange
4 ounces crumbled goat cheese
½ cup dried cranberries or other dried fruit
¼ cup toasted chopped walnuts (see Tip, page 99)
3 tablespoons chopped flat-leaf parsley
½ teaspoon coarse salt
¼ teaspoon freshly ground black pepper

This colorful salad includes a variety of textures and tastes. I like to serve this during the fall because of the autumnal flavors, but feel free to serve it year-round as a protein-packed side or main. With lots of good-quality protein, as well as omega-3 fatty acids via the walnuts, and antioxidants via the walnuts and cranberries, you can happily fill up on this gluten-free dish.

COOK THE QUINOA according to the package directions. Transfer to a medium bowl and let cool.

USING A ZESTER or rasplike tool, remove the zest from the orange and set aside. Cut off ½ inch from the top and bottom of the orange and set it on a cutting board. Using a sharp paring knife, slice off the outer peel in a downward motion, following the contour of the fruit. Work around the orange until all of the peel and pith is removed. While holding the fruit in one hand, cut out orange segments from between the membranes. Chop the segments and add them to the quinoa.

TO THE QUINOA, add the reserved orange zest, the goat cheese, cranberries, walnuts, parsley, salt, and pepper. Gently toss to combine.

TIP: Pronounced "KEEN-wah," quinoa is considered a grain because of the way it is eaten, but it is actually the seed of a plant native to Central America. It's often referred to as a superfood because it's packed with vitamins, minerals, protein, and fiber. Research suggests that it may have anti-inflammatory, heart health, and digestive health benefits—all great things for athletes.

SPINACH EGG DROP SOUP

SERVES 4

PER SERVING

CALORIES: 88.8
FAT: 2.7 g
SODIUM: 1,038.8 mg
CARBOHYDRATE: 6.5 g
FIBER: 1.8 g
SUGARS: 3.3 g
PROTEIN: 9.9 g

This incredibly easy soup takes minutes to whip up and will warm you through on chilly days. The key to getting the egg strands silky is to gently stir the soup while drizzling the eggs into the liquid. The eggs will quickly cook and leave behind cloudlike curds that are fun. While the eggs provide plenty of protein, I've included tofu for a heartier soup, and you can also add shredded cooked chicken.

4 cups vegetable or chicken broth
1¼-inch-thick slice fresh ginger (see Tip)
1 cup firm tofu, cut into cubes
4 large eggs
2 medium scallions (white and green parts), cut into 1-inch pieces
4 cups packed baby spinach
½ teaspoon freshly ground black pepper

IN A LARGE SAUCEPAN set over medium-low heat, bring the broth and ginger to a gentle simmer. Add the tofu.

IN A MEDIUM BOWL, beat the eggs with a fork or whisk.

USING ONE HAND, stir the broth in a circular motion. Slowly drizzle the eggs into the liquid as you continue to stir. Add the scallions and spinach, and cook until the spinach begins to wilt and the broth comes back to a simmer. Stir in the pepper and serve immediately.

TIP: Ginger has a pungent, spicy, and aromatic flavor, and can be used in various forms, including powdered, pickled, and fresh. It's most often used medicinally to relieve nausea and motion sickness, but it also has anti-inflammatory properties that are great for the athlete.

COLLARD GREENS
VEGETABLE ROLLS

MAKES 4 ROLLS

4 collard green
   leaves, stems
   removed
½ medium red bell
   pepper, cored,
   seeded, and cut
   into matchsticks
½ small English
   cucumber (about
   6 ounces), cut into
   matchsticks
½ medium ripe
   avocado, pitted
   and sliced
1 medium carrot,
   shredded
4 ounces cooked
   shredded chicken
   breast
Low-sodium soy
   sauce or tamari,
   for serving
   (optional)
Pickled ginger, for
   serving (optional)

A Southern staple, collard greens are an excellent source of vitamins A and C and folate, as well as a good source of calcium and fiber. While they're typically used in stews and hearty meals, I recently discovered that they make a great wrapper for vegetable rolls. This recipe is sort of like a cross between Vietnamese summer rolls and sushi, with colorful, crunchy vegetables wrapped up in collard green leaves.

FILL A LARGE POT halfway with water and bring to a boil over medium heat. Add the collard green leaves and cook, turning halfway through, until they are bright and flexible, 30 to 60 seconds. Using a slotted spoon, transfer the greens to a bowl of ice water and let cool. Drain, transfer to kitchen towels, and pat dry.

PLACE ONE LEAF on a work surface smooth side down. Close up the gap from where you removed the stem by slightly overlapping two sides of the leaf. Place a quarter of the bell pepper on the bottom quarter of the leaf, with the matchsticks placed horizontally across the leaf. Top with a quarter of the cucumber, avocado, carrot, and chicken. Pull the bottom of the leaf up over the vegetables and chicken, and then roll the leaf up, tucking in the sides as you go to keep the filling inside. Trim any excess leaf from the end. Repeat with the remaining ingredients.

TO SERVE, cut each roll in half and serve with soy sauce and ginger (if using).

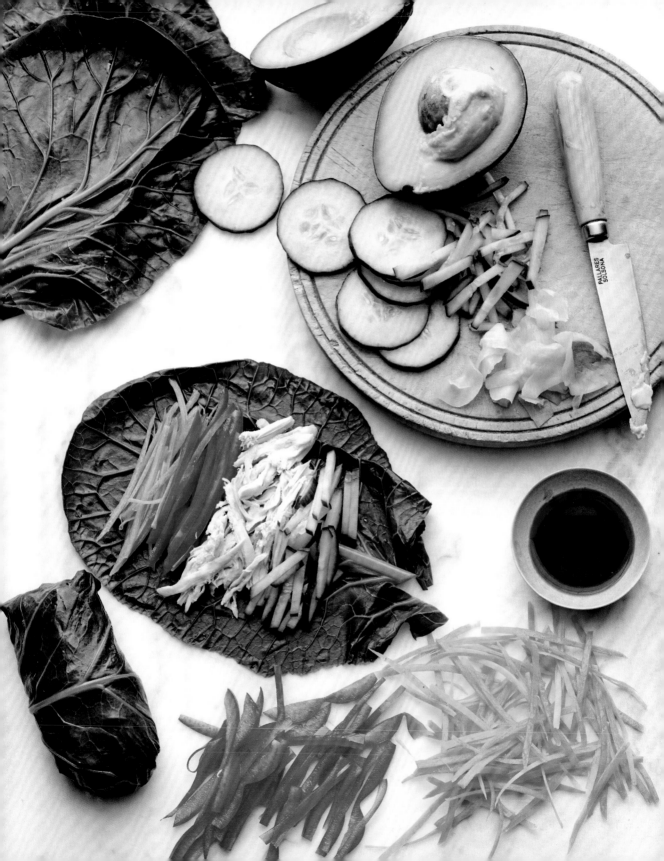

PER SERVING

CALORIES: 331.2
FAT: 9.4 g
SODIUM: 1,045.1 mg
CARBOHYDRATE: 35.5 g
FIBER: 4.5 g
SUGARS: 1.7 g
PROTEIN: 26.8 g

CHICKEN, QUINOA, AND
VEGETABLE SOUP

SERVES 4

3 teaspoons extra-
  virgin olive oil
1 medium onion,
  chopped
2 garlic cloves,
  chopped
2 medium celery
  stalks, chopped
1 medium carrot,
  chopped
1 cup quinoa
4 cups chicken broth
2 tablespoons
  chopped fresh dill
2 cups shredded or
  chopped cooked
  chicken

Although most grains are not a core food (see page 18), quinoa is okay, because it isn't actually a grain. This recipe is like a version of traditional chicken noodle soup, only instead of noodles, it has quinoa for texture and a boost of protein. The quinoa also adds a fair amount of fiber—something that plain white noodles lack—and, as discussed throughout this book (see pages 20 and 75), fiber helps dilute the blood sugar response of any of the grains we eat!

IN A MEDIUM SAUCEPAN set over medium-high heat, heat the oil. When the oil begins to shimmer, add the onion, garlic, celery, and carrot. Cook, stirring, until slightly soft, about 5 minutes. Stir in the quinoa and cook until slightly toasted, 1 to 2 minutes. Add the chicken broth and 1½ cups water. Bring to a boil. Reduce the heat to low, partially cover, and simmer until the quinoa is soft, 10 minutes.

STIR IN THE DILL AND CHICKEN. Serve hot.

MANHATTAN-STYLE
FISH CHOWDER

SERVES 4

Although I am from the Boston area, where creamy white chowders reign, I have to admit that the tomato-based versions are superior when it comes to nutrition and performance. Tomatoes contain lycopene, which has many health benefits (see Tip). Here, we replaced starchy potatoes—typical in New England–style chowders—with cauliflower for extra fiber and nutrients, and used lean Canadian bacon for its smoky flavor.

IN A MEDIUM SAUCEPAN set over medium-high heat, heat the oil. When the oil begins to shimmer, add the onion, bacon, celery, and carrots. Cook, stirring, until soft, 5 minutes. Add the thyme and cook for 1 minute. Stir in the tomato paste and cook for 1 more minute. Add the broth, diced tomatoes, and cauliflower. Bring to a boil, reduce the heat to low, and simmer until the cauliflower is tender, 7 to 10 minutes.

ADD THE FISH TO THE POT. Cover and cook until the fish is opaque, 3 to 5 minutes. Turn off the heat, stir in the pepper and parsley, and serve.

TIP: Preliminary research shows that lycopene, an antioxidant that gives tomatoes their red color, may help prevent cell damage, aging, and chronic disease. Cooking tomatoes actually makes the phytonutrient more available to be absorbed by the body, as does combining them with fats.

1 tablespoon extra-virgin olive oil
½ medium onion, chopped
3 slices Canadian bacon, chopped (about 2 ounces)
2 medium celery stalks, chopped
2 small carrots, chopped
½ teaspoon dried thyme
1 tablespoon tomato paste
2 cups seafood broth
½ cup canned diced tomatoes
1½ cups cauliflower florets
¾ pound firm white fish like cod or halibut, cut into small pieces
Pinch of freshly ground black pepper
¼ cup chopped fresh flat-leaf parsley

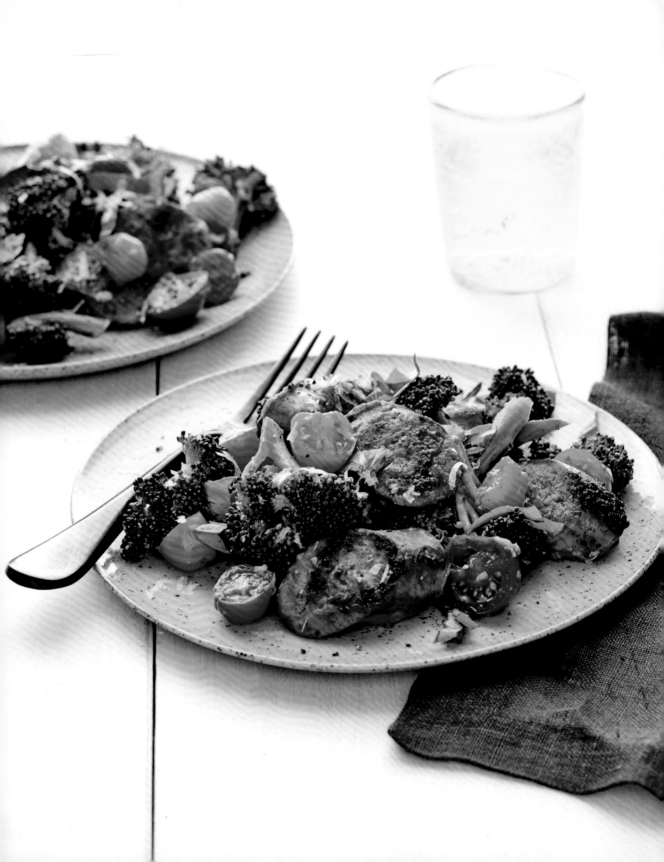

TURKEY SAUSAGE
WITH BROCCOLI AND TOMATOES

SERVES 4

PER SERVING

CALORIES: 246.3
FAT: 10.3 g
SODIUM: 928.5 mg
CARBOHYDRATE: 21.1 g
FIBER: 4.6 g
SUGARS: 5.7 g
PROTEIN: 21.1 g

This quick, healthy, and vibrantly colored dish is a standard in my house. The broccoli, tomatoes, and basil provide dietary fiber and vitamins A and C, and the turkey adds a hefty dose of satiating protein. Feel free to use chicken sausage, and you can opt for mild if you don't like too much spicy heat.

Bunch of broccoli, trimmed and cut into florets (about 1¼ pounds)
Canola or olive oil cooking spray
4 hot Italian turkey sausage links (about 13 ounces)
1 pint grape tomatoes, halved
½ cup chopped fresh basil leaves
¼ cup grated Romano cheese (see Tip)

STEAM THE BROCCOLI in a large pot fitted with a steamer basket set over medium-high heat until the florets are bright green and the stems can be pierced with a knife, 3 to 5 minutes. Set aside.

SPRAY A LARGE NONSTICK SKILLET or sauté pan with cooking spray and set it over medium heat. Add the sausage and cook until browned on all sides, about 7 minutes. Remove the sausage from the pan and cut into ½-inch slices. Return the slices to the pan and cook until they're no longer pink, 1 to 2 minutes per side. Add the tomatoes and cook until they begin to soften, 3 to 5 minutes. Gently stir in the broccoli and 1 to 2 tablespoons water. Scrape up the flavorful bits on the bottom of the pan. Stir in the basil and cheese. Remove the pan from the heat and serve hot.

TIP: Cheese is packed with protein and calcium but is often loaded with unwanted saturated fat. As a healthy compromise, use small amounts of intensely flavored cheeses like Parmesan, Romano, and sharp Cheddar.

PER SERVING

CALORIES: 246.7
FAT: 3.7 g
SODIUM: 680.1 mg
CARBOHYDRATE: 42.9 g
FIBER: 10 g
SUGARS: 2.3 g
PROTEIN: 14.1 g

KALE SOUP
WITH WHITE BEANS AND TOMATOES
SERVES 6

- 1 tablespoon canola oil
- 8 large garlic cloves, minced
- 1 medium yellow onion, chopped
- 2 teaspoons no-sodium-added Italian herb seasoning
- 2 medium plum tomatoes, chopped
- 2 (15-ounce) cans cannellini, navy, or other white beans
- 4 cups vegetable or chicken broth
- 6 cups chopped kale (see Tip)
- ½ teaspoon freshly ground black pepper
- ¼ cup chopped fresh flat-leaf parsley, for garnish

This is one of my favorite recipes for those cooler days after training outside, though it can really be enjoyed any time of the year. Soups are generally a good recovery drink option, because of their higher sodium content. Blending half the beans with the broth and stirring the mixture into the soup help thicken the dish without adding extra fat, such as cream. This recipe makes a moderate-size batch, so you can store it in the refrigerator or freezer for future meals.

IN A LARGE POT set over medium heat, heat the oil. When the oil begins to shimmer, add the garlic and onion and cook, stirring, until soft, 3 to 5 minutes. Add the herb seasoning and cook, stirring, until soft, 1 to 2 minutes. Stir in the tomatoes, 1 can of the beans, and 3 cups of the broth. Bring to a boil, cover, and simmer for 5 minutes.

MEANWHILE, put the remaining can of beans and 1 cup of the broth into a blender or food processor. Blend until smooth. Stir the mixture into the soup and simmer, covered, for another 5 to 10 minutes. Add the kale and pepper and stir to combine. Cover and bring to a boil. Turn off the heat and let cool for 3 to 5 minutes before serving.

TO SERVE, ladle the soup into six bowls and garnish with the parsley.

TIP: Kale is a wonderful member of the cabbage family and is rich in nutrients like iron; vitamins A, C, and K; and calcium. While you can get kale year-round, you'll often find more varieties of kale in the fall and winter, when it's in season. Use whatever kind you like—whether curly, purple, or lacinato—for this dish.

SLOW-COOKER TURKEY CHILI

SERVES 15

PER SERVING

CALORIES: 261.4
FAT: 9 g
SODIUM: 864.3 mg
CARBOHYDRATE: 22.2 g
FIBER: 8.2 g
SUGARS: 2.7 g
PROTEIN: 24 g

Packed with nutrients like vitamins A and C, protein, and dietary fiber, and spiked with flavorful aromatics, herbs, and spices, this hearty dish is a perfect meal to follow long training days during the winter months. Make a batch for a crowd or for a few days of eating, or simply freeze the leftovers for later (see Tip). This is a core foods favorite and can be the perfect go-to during the week after making a batch Sunday afternoon.

SPRAY THE INSIDE of a large 6-quart slow cooker with cooking spray.

IN A LARGE SKILLET or sauté pan set over medium-high heat, heat the canola oil. When the oil begins to shimmer, add the onions and garlic, and cook until soft, about 5 minutes. Add the chili powder, oregano, cumin, paprika, salt, and black pepper. Cook until the spices are fragrant, about 2 minutes. Transfer the mixture to the slow cooker.

USING THE SAME PAN set over medium heat, cook the ground turkey in batches until browned, draining the excess liquid, if necessary. Transfer the turkey to the slow cooker. Add the bell peppers, diced tomatoes, tomato paste, and vinegar. Add 2 cups of water and the beans. Stir well.

COVER AND COOK on low for 6 hours or high for 3 hours. Stir well before serving.

TIP: To save on precious space in the freezer, pour leftover chili into resealable freezer bags. Press out all the air, seal the bags, and place them flat in the freezer. Once frozen, the bags can be stacked or arranged upright. It's much easier than playing freezer Jenga with plastic containers.

Canola oil cooking spray
2 tablespoons canola oil
2 medium onions, chopped
6 garlic cloves, minced
¼ cup chili powder
1½ tablespoons dried oregano
1½ tablespoons ground cumin
1 tablespoon paprika
2 teaspoons coarse salt
½ teaspoon freshly ground black pepper
3 pounds lean ground turkey
1 medium red bell pepper, seeded and chopped
1 medium green bell pepper, seeded and chopped
1 medium yellow bell pepper, seeded and chopped
2 (14-ounce) cans diced tomatoes
1 (6-ounce) can tomato paste
3 tablespoons red wine vinegar
3 (15- or 16-ounce) cans beans, drained and rinsed (use black, pinto, kidney, or whatever you like)

QUINOA-CRUSTED
CHICKEN TENDERS

SERVES 4

1 cup cooked quinoa
½ cup shredded
    Parmesan cheese
1 teaspoon dried
    thyme
1 teaspoon coarse
    salt
2 large eggs
1 pound chicken
    tenders
Olive oil cooking
    spray

These crunchy tenders pack a double protein punch, thanks to the quinoa and chicken. Delicious on their own, they're fantastic served with dips like ketchup, blue cheese dressing, or mustard. Small amounts of noncore condiments are perfectly fine! The tenders might taste like fast food, but they're a lot healthier and fall within the requirements of the core foods. If you can't find chicken tenders at the store, buy a boneless, skinless chicken breast and cut it into strips.

PREHEAT THE OVEN to 300°F.

ON A RIMMED BAKING SHEET, spread the quinoa in a thin layer. Bake until toasted, about 30 minutes. Let cool. Transfer to a large bowl and stir in the Parmesan, thyme, and salt.

RAISE THE HEAT to 425°F. Line the baking sheet with parchment paper.

IN A SHALLOW BOWL, beat the eggs together. Dip the chicken pieces in the egg, and then roll them in the quinoa mixture. Place the pieces on the prepared baking sheet and spritz with cooking spray.

BAKE THE CHICKEN until it is cooked through, 15 to 20 minutes. Serve immediately.

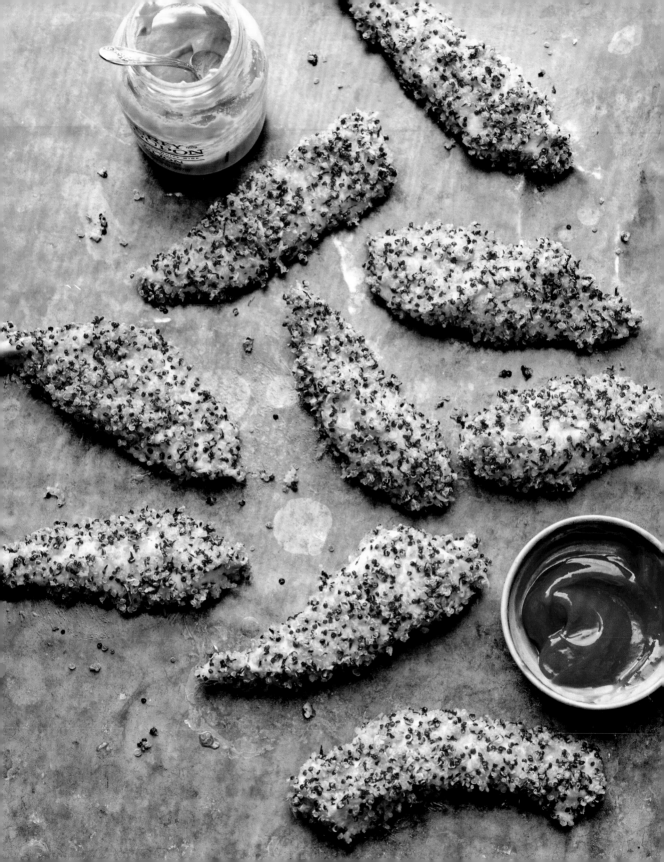

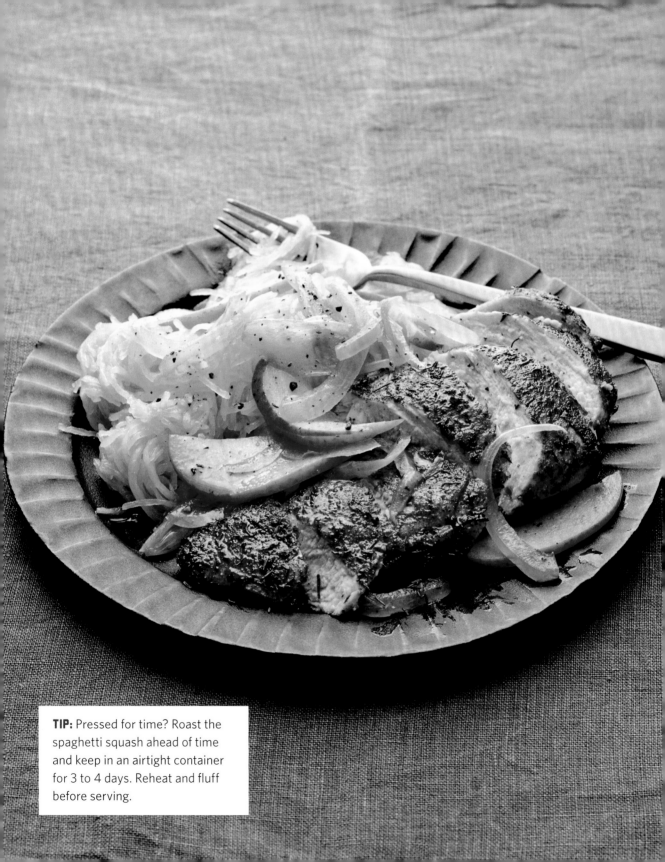

TIP: Pressed for time? Roast the spaghetti squash ahead of time and keep in an airtight container for 3 to 4 days. Reheat and fluff before serving.

SAGE-RUBBED
CHICKEN BREAST
WITH SPAGHETTI SQUASH

SERVES 4

PER SERVING

CALORIES: 351.3
FAT: 15.7 g
SODIUM: 867.3 mg
CARBOHYDRATE: 21.3 g
FIBER: 3.5 g
SUGARS: 8.7 g
PROTEIN: 32.7 g

Low in calories and carbohydrates, spaghetti squash has a mild flavor, and when cooked, its flesh separates into noodlelike strands. I like using it as a substitute when a recipe calls for regular spaghetti, which should really be enjoyed in evenings as a replenishment meal only once a week, the night before the week's longest and hardest workout.

1 small to medium spaghetti squash (about 1 pound)
3 tablespoons canola or olive oil
1½ teaspoons ground sage
1 teaspoon garlic powder
½ teaspoon dried thyme
1¼ teaspoons coarse salt
4 boneless, skinless chicken breasts (1 to 1¼ pounds)
1 medium onion, thinly sliced
1 large apple, thinly sliced
½ cup unsweetened apple juice
½ cup chicken broth
1 tablespoon apple cider vinegar
½ teaspoon freshly ground black pepper

PREHEAT THE OVEN to 400°F.

USING A SHARP KNIFE, carefully slice the squash in half lengthwise. Remove the seeds and discard. Rub 1 tablespoon of the oil over the squash and place it cut side down on a baking sheet. Roast until a knife can be easily inserted into the squash, 30 to 45 minutes (see Tip, opposite). Remove from the oven and let cool.

IN A SMALL BOWL, combine the sage, garlic powder, thyme, and ¼ teaspoon of the salt. Rub the mixture all over the chicken breasts. In a large nonstick sauté pan set over medium-high heat, heat the remaining 2 tablespoons oil. Add the chicken and cook until browned on both sides, about 3 minutes per side. Transfer to a plate. Add the onion and apple to the pan and cook until slightly soft, 2 to 3 minutes. Add the apple juice, broth, and vinegar and simmer for about 1 minute. Add the chicken, along with any juices, back to the pan. Cover and cook until the chicken is cooked through, about 5 minutes. Season with the remaining 1 teaspoon salt and the pepper.

USING A FORK, scrape the insides of the spaghetti squash and pile the spaghetti-like noodles onto a serving platter. Top with the chicken and juices, and serve.

SALMON PATTIES
OVER FIELD GREENS

MAKES 4 PATTIES

1 (14.75-ounce) can salmon, well drained, picked through for bones and skin

½ cup finely chopped red onion

¼ cup chopped fresh flat-leaf parsley

2 tablespoons chopped fresh basil

2 tablespoons fresh lemon juice

1 teaspoon grated lemon zest

2 large eggs

2 tablespoons canola or olive oil

1 (7-ounce) package of field green salad mix

Lemon wedges, for serving

Canned salmon is relatively inexpensive and a great shelf-stable source of omega-3 fatty acids. While salmon steaks and fillets are optimal for certain dishes, I find canned perfect for making patties and burgers, as it is already cooked and ready to use. Concerned about PCBs (polychlorinated biphenyls), the dioxins found in farmed salmon? Look for canned salmon that's labeled "wild-caught," Alaskan pink, or sockeye.

IN A MEDIUM BOWL, using a fork, break up the salmon into small to medium flakes. Add the onion, parsley, basil, lemon juice, lemon zest, and eggs. Stir well. Divide the mixture into equal quarters and form each into patties that are about 1 inch thick. Place on a baking sheet lined with waxed or parchment paper. Refrigerate for at least 30 minutes.

IN A LARGE NONSTICK SAUTÉ PAN set over medium-high heat, heat the oil. When the oil begins to shimmer, gently place the patties in the pan. Cook until browned on both sides, about 2 minutes per side.

DIVIDE THE GREENS among four serving plates. Serve the burgers on top of the greens (see Tip), with lemon wedges.

TIP: If you want to eat the patties in burgerlike fashion, use sturdy lettuce leaves, like romaine, to form a bun. You can also use a core-ratio-friendly grain product such as Joseph's brand Flax, Oat Bran & Whole Wheat Flour Tortillas to wrap your burgers.

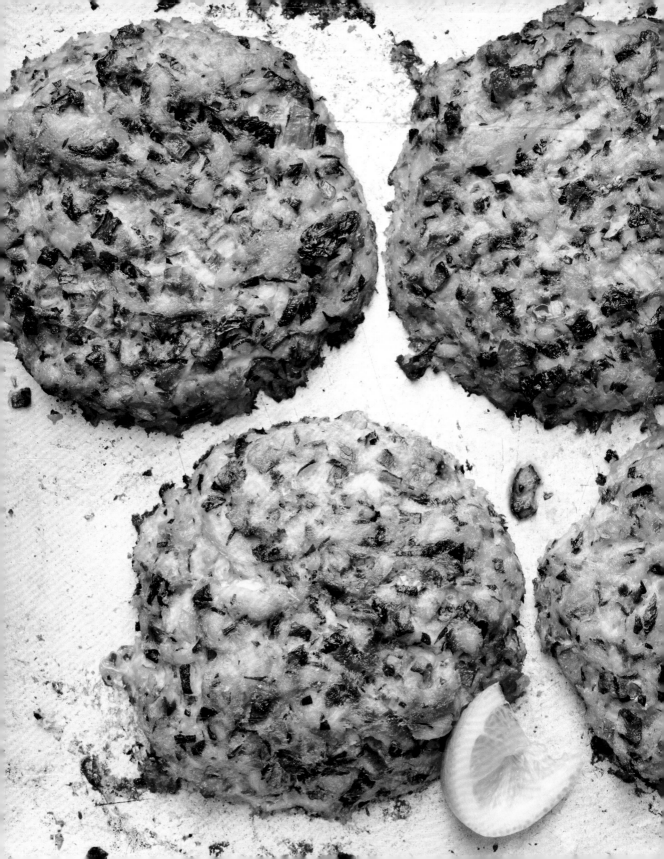

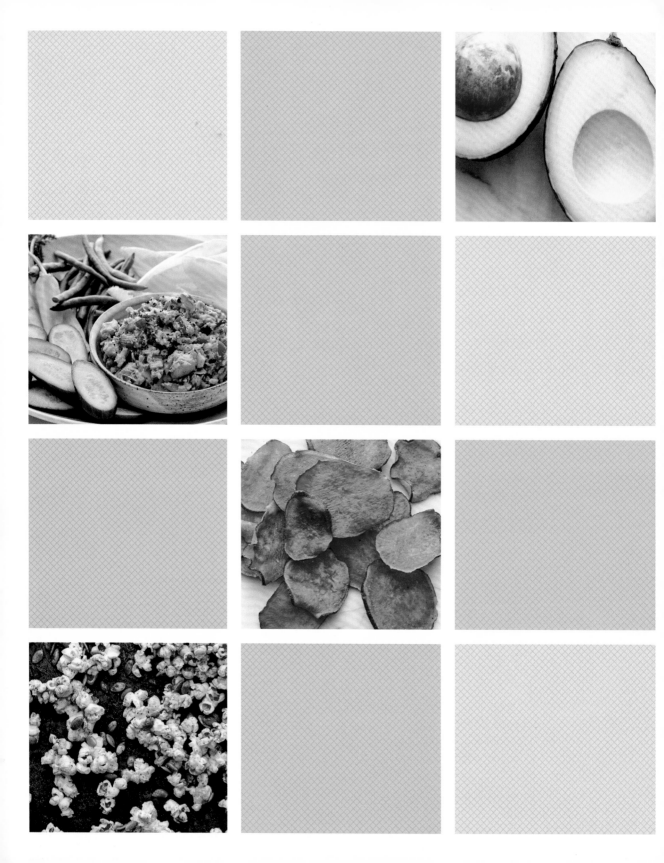

SNACKS

ORANGE-INFUSED
YOGURT PARFAIT WITH
BLUEBERRIES

144

HERBED
COTTAGE CHEESE

145

EDAMAME-
AVOCADO DIP

146

BLACK BEAN
CILANTRO DIP

148

APPLE, CELERY,
AND RAISIN SALAD

149

GUACAMOLE WITH
TOASTED SPICES

151

CHILI-SPICED
POPCORN WITH
PUMPKIN SEEDS

152

WALNUT-STUFFED
DATES

154

FRUIT AND NUT
ENERGY BLEND

155

BAKED SWEET
POTATO CHIPS

156

ORANGE-INFUSED
YOGURT PARFAIT
WITH BLUEBERRIES

SERVES 4

- **4 small navel oranges (see Tip)**
- **1 cup fresh or frozen blueberries**
- **2 cups nonfat Greek yogurt, such as Fage**
- **¼ teaspoon vanilla extract**
- **2 teaspoons honey**

Yogurt is a delicious food that's packed with protein and calcium. But if you've ever looked at the nutrition facts label of some flavored yogurts, you'll notice that they're typically loaded with sugar. In fact, a 6-ounce container of a popular brand of blueberry yogurt contains 24 grams of sugar and has a core ratio of 3 (higher than the recommended 2). To take advantage of the benefits of yogurt without all that added sugar, I like to pile naturally sweet fruit on top of plain yogurt and add just a touch of honey.

USING A ZESTER or rasplike tool, remove about ½ teaspoon of zest from the oranges while avoiding the bitter white pith; set aside. Cut off ¼ inch from the top and bottom of the fruit. Using a sharp paring knife, cut the peel away from the orange, following the contours of the fruit. While holding an orange in one hand, cut between the membranes to remove the segments, dropping the segments into a medium bowl. Squeeze the juices from the membranes into the bowl. Add the blueberries and toss together.

IN A MEDIUM BOWL, combine the reserved orange zest, the yogurt, vanilla, and ¼ cup of the juice from the orange-and-blueberry mixture. Mix well.

IN FOUR 6-OUNCE SERVING CUPS, place ¼ cup of the orange-and-blueberry mixture in the bottoms. Top with ½ cup yogurt and another ¼-cup layer of fruit. Drizzle ½ teaspoon honey on top. Serve.

TIP: If you're concerned about pesticides that may coat the aromatic peel of conventionally grown citrus fruit, look for organic varieties, which don't contain the pesticides.

HERBED
COTTAGE CHEESE

SERVES 4

PER SERVING

CALORIES: 81.5
FAT: 1.2 g
SODIUM: 459 mg
CARBOHYDRATE: 3 g
FIBER: 0 g
SUGARS: 3.1 g
PROTEIN: 14 g

Fresh herbs add great flavor to dishes without contributing excess sodium, fat, or sugar. And herbs are delicious when paired with soft cheeses like goat cheese and, as in this recipe, cottage cheese. Serve this green-flecked cottage cheese with fresh crudités like carrots, red bell peppers, cucumbers, and celery, or with core-ratio-friendly chips (see Tip).

2 cups nonfat or 1% cottage cheese
2 tablespoons mixed chopped fresh herbs, such as parsley, chives, or dill
¼ teaspoon freshly ground black pepper
Freshly cut vegetables, such as carrots, red bell peppers, and cucumbers, for serving (optional)
Crackers, for serving (optional)

IN A MEDIUM BOWL, stir the cottage cheese and herbs together. Season with pepper. Transfer to a serving dish, and serve with vegetables and crackers (if using).

TIP: Grains are generally not part of the core diet when eaten outside the workout windows, but I occasionally find some products that can work well if they meet the core ratio requirements (see page 20). Bean-based chips and snacks like Way Better Chips or Beanitos are great core-ratio-friendly accompaniments to this dip. Just watch your portion size and make sure the flavor you choose meets the core ratio.

EDAMAME-AVOCADO DIP

MAKES 2½ CUPS; SERVES 10

12 ounces frozen shelled edamame, thawed (see Tip)
1 large ripe avocado, pitted and peeled
2 garlic cloves
¼ cup fresh lemon juice
¼ cup extra-virgin olive oil
1¼ teaspoons coarse salt
½ teaspoon freshly ground black pepper
1 teaspoon ground cumin

Often found salted and in fuzzy pods in Japanese restaurants, edamame (or soybeans) are a protein-rich food. Their soft, beanlike texture is delicious and versatile. In this recipe, I blend the thawed, shelled beans with avocado to make a tasty, green-hued dip that's packed with an ideal mix of protein, fat, and fiber. It's great served with vegetables and chips for dipping, or try using it as a sandwich spread.

IN A FOOD PROCESSOR OR BLENDER, combine the edamame, avocado, garlic, lemon juice, olive oil, salt, pepper, and cumin. Blend until smooth, adding up to ¼ cup water if the mixture seems too thick.

TIP: Edamame is the only vegetable that contains all nine essential amino acids (the ones your body cannot create), making it a complete protein. Try substituting these beans in recipes that call for green peas or lima beans.

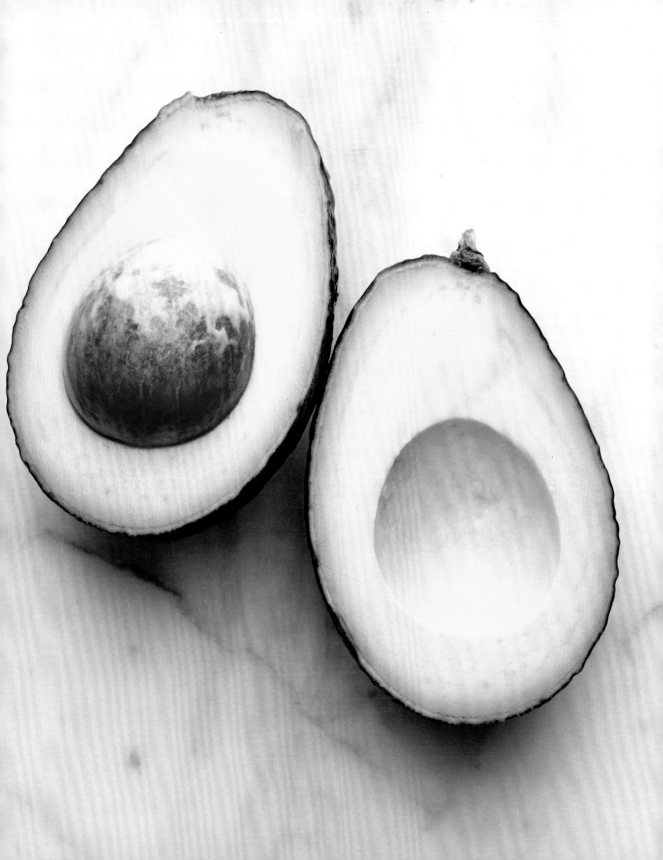

BLACK BEAN CILANTRO DIP

MAKES 1½ CUPS; SERVES 12

1 (15-ounce) can
   black beans
1 teaspoon canola oil
5 to 6 cherry
   tomatoes, halved
   (about ⅓ cup)
¼ medium red onion,
   chopped
1 garlic clove,
   chopped
½ medium jalapeño
   pepper, cored,
   seeded, and
   chopped
½ teaspoon ground
   cumin
2 tablespoons
   chopped fresh
   cilantro leaves
   and stems
2 teaspoons fresh
   lime juice
¼ teaspoon coarse
   salt

Rich and creamy, this black bean dip can be whipped up in minutes. A healthy alternative to cheesy and fat-laden dips—it provides plenty of protein, dietary fiber, and iron—it's great to serve at a get-together. Bring it to the party with core-ratio-friendly chips (see page 156) or serve with raw vegetables. This dip has a subtle note of heat from the jalapeño (see Tip), and you can leave it out if you prefer a milder flavor.

DRAIN THE BLACK BEANS in a strainer set over a bowl; reserve the liquid.

IN A MEDIUM SAUTÉ PAN set over medium heat, heat the oil. When the oil begins to shimmer, add the tomatoes, onion, garlic, and jalapeño. Cook, stirring, until soft, about 5 minutes. Add the cumin and cook for about 1 minute, until fragrant. Transfer the mixture to the bowl of a food processor. Add the beans along with 2 tablespoons of the reserved bean liquid and the cilantro to the food processor and puree until smooth. Add the lime juice and salt, and puree again.

THE DIP WILL KEEP in an airtight container in the refrigerator for 2 to 3 days.

TIP: Contrary to popular belief, the heat in a chili pepper does not come from the seeds. Capsaicin, the compound that makes our ears ring and mouth burn, is actually concentrated in the white membrane of the pepper that the seeds cling to. So if you want to reduce or increase the heat of a dish, remove or keep the membranes.

APPLE, CELERY, AND RAISIN
SALAD

SERVES 4

PER SERVING

CALORIES: 160.5
FAT: 5.9 g
SODIUM: 23.3 mg
CARBOHYDRATE: 26.1 g
FIBER: 3.6 g
SUGARS: 19.2 g
PROTEIN: 4.6 g

Bored with your snack routine of plain fruit? This refreshing salad will keep you full and energized with its balance of carbohydrates, fat, and protein. It also provides different textures, from crispy to chewy, to keep things interesting and satisfying. By including walnuts, we are also promoting our all-important omega-3 campaign. I enjoy using a mix of apples, such as Honeycrisp, Mutsu, and Gala, for a variety of taste, color, and texture—and be sure to keep the skin on to get fiber and vitamin C (just don't eat this too close to a run workout!).

2 medium to large apples, cored and chopped into bite-size pieces
1 medium celery stalk, chopped
¼ cup raisins
½ cup 2% Greek yogurt, such as Fage
½ teaspoon honey
Pinch of ground cinnamon
¼ cup toasted chopped walnuts

IN A LARGE BOWL, combine the apples, celery, raisins, yogurt, honey, and cinnamon. Fold all the ingredients together until well combined. Cover and refrigerate for at least 1 hour. Sprinkle the walnuts on top before serving.

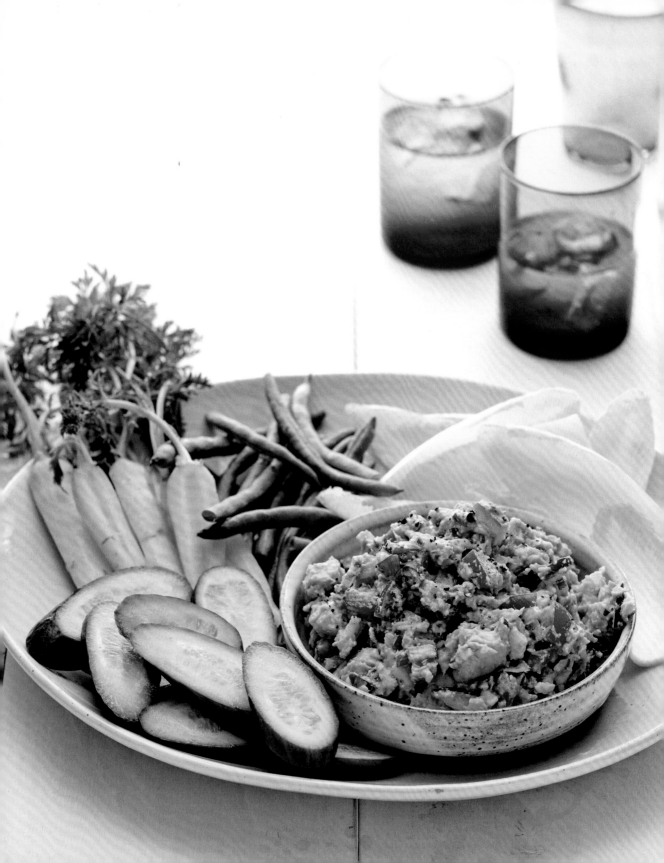

GUACAMOLE
WITH TOASTED SPICES

MAKES 2 CUPS; SERVES 8

PER SERVING

CALORIES: 81.5
FAT: 11.8 g
SODIUM: 71.8 mg
CARBOHYDRATE: 4.8 g
FIBER: 3.1 g
SUGARS: 0.2 g
PROTEIN: 1 g

Creamy and rich, avocados are a great source of monounsaturated fat (ALA, the omega-3 fatty acid that is a precursor to EPA/DHA), the heart-healthy kind that helps lower cholesterol. I love that the health benefits of avocados mean that guacamole—one of the most delicious dips ever—can be considered a superfood (depending on what you eat it with!). Serve it as a quick snack with raw veggies or core-ratio-friendly chips (see page 156), or use it as a spread for sandwiches. It's also fantastic with Chipotle Chicken Tacos (page 173).

- 1 teaspoon ground cumin
- ¼ teaspoon cayenne pepper
- 2 large ripe Hass avocados, pitted and peeled (see Tip)
- ½ small red onion, finely chopped
- 1 large plum tomato, seeded and chopped
- ¼ cup chopped fresh cilantro leaves
- 2 tablespoons fresh lime juice
- ½ teaspoon coarse salt
- 1 teaspoon extra-virgin olive oil

IN A SMALL SAUTÉ PAN set over low heat, toast the cumin and cayenne, constantly shaking the pan or stirring the spices to prevent burning, until fragrant, about 5 minutes. Transfer the spices to a small bowl and let cool.

IN A MEDIUM BOWL, combine the avocados, onion, tomato, and cilantro. Add the toasted cumin and cayenne, lime juice, salt, and oil. Stir gently. The guacamole is best served immediately, though it will keep in the refrigerator for about a day.

> **TIP:** The best way to ripen an avocado is to place it in a paper bag with other ripe fruits such as apples and bananas. These ripe fruits will naturally give off ethylene gas, which in turn hastens the ripening process in an avocado. Once ripe, store away from ripe fruit for 2 to 3 days at room temperature.

CHILI-SPICED POPCORN
WITH PUMPKIN SEEDS

MAKES ABOUT 2 QUARTS: SERVES 4

- 2 tablespoons canola oil
- ¼ cup popcorn kernels
- 2 tablespoons light butter (see Tip, page 103)
- ¼ cup honey
- ¼ teaspoon cayenne pepper
- ¼ teaspoon chili powder
- ¼ teaspoon coarse salt
- ½ cup toasted shelled pumpkin seeds (see Tip, page 99)

Sure, popcorn may get a bad rap because of all the sodium and fat that's added to it (movie theater popcorn!), but it can be a nutritious snack packed with dietary fiber, antioxidants, vitamins, and minerals. I like to pop dry kernels in a little oil on the stovetop, but if you want to minimize your fat intake while on a fat-losing objective, you can use air-popped popcorn, too. Although popcorn on its own is typically considered a high-glycemic grain (like pasta), when combined with fats and fibers, as it is in this recipe, it can become a nutritious snack—one with a reasonable blood sugar response.

PREHEAT THE OVEN to 300°F. Line rimmed baking sheet pans with parchment paper.

IN A LARGE POT set over medium-high heat, heat the oil. When the oil begins to shimmer, toss in 2 to 3 kernels of popcorn, and cover with a tight-fitting lid. Once a kernel pops, add the remaining kernels. Cover and gently shake the pan so that the kernels are in a single layer and get coated with the oil. When the kernels begin to pop, gently shake the pan. If possible, keep the lid slightly ajar so that steam can escape, but be careful of spattering oil and high-flying popcorn. Once the popping slows down, after about 3 minutes, or when the popping is separated by more than 2 seconds, remove the pan from the heat and transfer the popcorn to a bowl.

RETURN THE PAN to the stove and set it over medium-low heat. Add the butter, honey, cayenne, chili powder, and salt. Bring the mixture to a simmer, and cook until slightly thickened, 1 to 2 minutes. Add the pumpkin seeds and popcorn, and gently fold the mixture until the popcorn and seeds are coated with the honey mixture. Transfer the mixture to the prepared baking sheets and spread into a single layer.

BAKE, stirring once or twice, until golden, about 15 minutes. Let cool before eating. The popcorn will keep in an airtight container for 2 to 3 days.

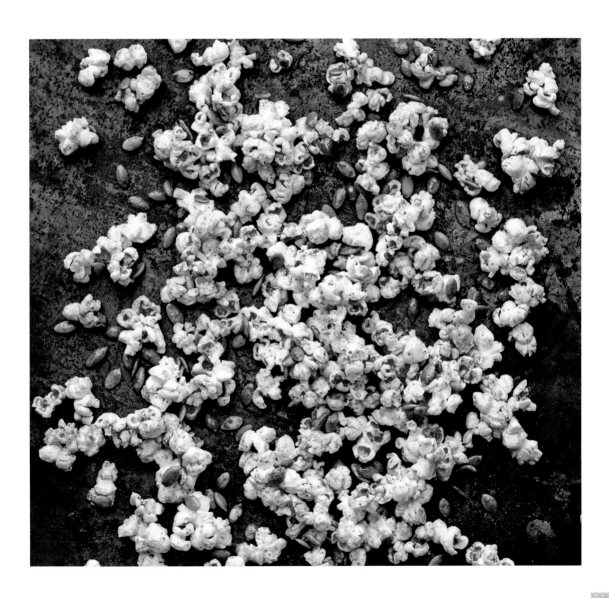

PER SERVING

CALORIES: 188
FAT: 5.4 g
SODIUM: 20.2 mg
CARBOHYDRATE: 36.9 g
FIBER: 3.6 g
SUGARS: 32.1 g
PROTEIN: 2.8 g

WALNUT-STUFFED DATES

MAKES 16 STUFFED DATES; SERVES 8

- 8 to 12 ounces (about 16) medjool dates with pits
- ½ cup walnut halves, broken in half
- 8 teaspoons soft goat cheese

These stuffed dates work great as a snack, packed with fiber, protein, fat, and a touch of sweetness. Dates also provide a great dose of potassium, a key electrolyte for endurance athletes, and one in which athletes with higher sweat rates may be deficient. These dates are calorie dense and satiating, making them ideal for heavy training weeks when caloric burns are high and you are eating between workouts in core periods. To make these a portable, go-anywhere snack, omit the goat cheese.

USING A PARING KNIFE, cut a vertical slit in the dates and remove the pits. Stuff the dates with pieces of walnut. Then stuff with the goat cheese.

FRUIT AND NUT ENERGY BLEND

MAKES 5 CUPS; SERVES 15

Nuts are a great source of protein, good fats, and micronutrients, so I made this special blend to maximize the vitamins, minerals, and fats available through each nut. Eating a serving of this blend each day will help get your fat and protein intake up, which will support tissue repair and enhance nutrient absorption by the gut. For those of you who are looking to gain muscle and maintain weight, eat this mixture daily. It's a win-win to get added caloric density, along with the nutrient density nuts offer. Choose raw or toasted nuts, per your tastes.

½ cup unsalted macadamia nuts
1½ cups walnut halves
1 cup unsalted almonds
½ cup unsalted Brazil nuts
1 cup unsalted sunflower seeds
1¼ cups dried cherries or chopped dates
1 cup toasted unsweetened coconut flakes (see Tip)

IN A LARGE BOWL, combine the macadamia nuts, walnuts, almonds, Brazil nuts, sunflower seeds, dried cherries, and coconut flakes. The blend will keep in an airtight container for 2 to 3 months.

TIP: Toasted coconut adds a light and crispy texture and warm, tropical flavor to this blend. To keep the recipe core-ratio-friendly and avoid added sugars, I like unsweetened coconut flakes, which you can buy in most supermarkets or health food stores. To toast, spread out the coconut into a thin layer on a baking sheet. Bake in a 350°F. oven for 5 to 10 minutes, or until golden and crisp.

PER SERVING

CALORIES: 260.3
FAT: 14.4 g
SODIUM: 286.9 mg
CARBOHYDRATE: 31.6 g
FIBER: 3.9 g
SUGARS: 0 g
PROTEIN: 2.1 g

BAKED SWEET POTATO CHIPS

SERVES 2

2 tablespoons canola
oil, plus more for
the baking sheets
2 medium or large
sweet potatoes,
washed and
scrubbed
½ teaspoons adobo
seasoning
½ teaspoon coarse
salt

Sweet potatoes are one of the most nutritious foods you can eat—and they are so versatile! Unlike russet potatoes or red potatoes, the sweet varieties raise blood sugar at a slower rate. Not to mention they are packed with nutrients like beta-carotene, vitamins C and E, and dietary fiber. This recipe is the easiest and possibly best-tasting way I know to prepare this root vegetable. The thin slices crisp up in the oven and taste just like they were fried, but they really weren't!

PREHEAT THE OVEN to 375°F. Lightly oil a few baking sheets.

USING A SHARP KNIFE or mandoline (be very careful!), slice the potatoes into ⅛-inch-thick slices. In a large bowl, toss the slices with the oil, adobo, and salt. Arrange the slices in a single layer on the prepared baking sheets.

BAKE FOR 15 MINUTES. Flip the slices over and bake until the slices are golden in spots, 10 to 15 more minutes. Let cool for 5 minutes to crisp up.

THE COOLED CHIPS are best eaten right away, but they will keep in an airtight container for 2 to 3 days.

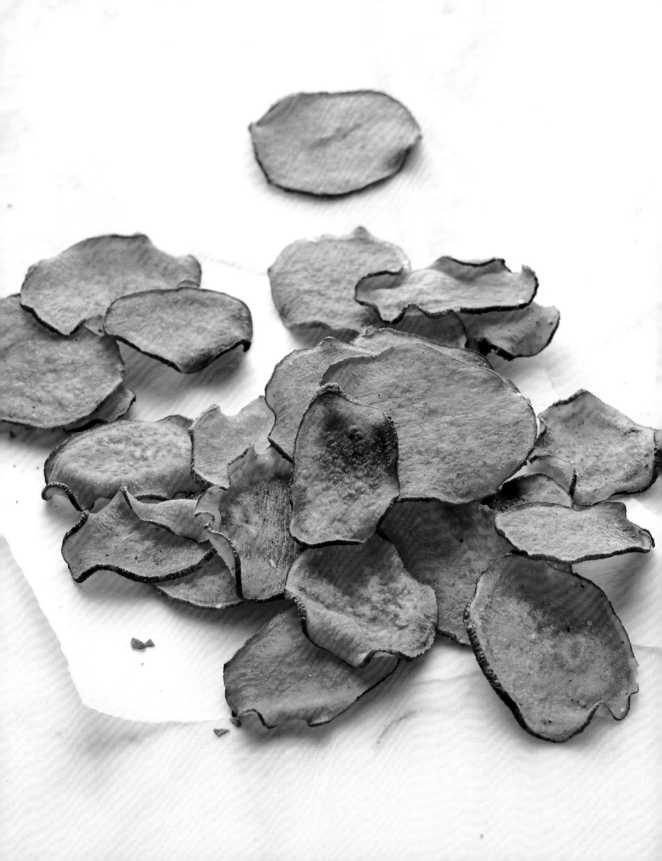

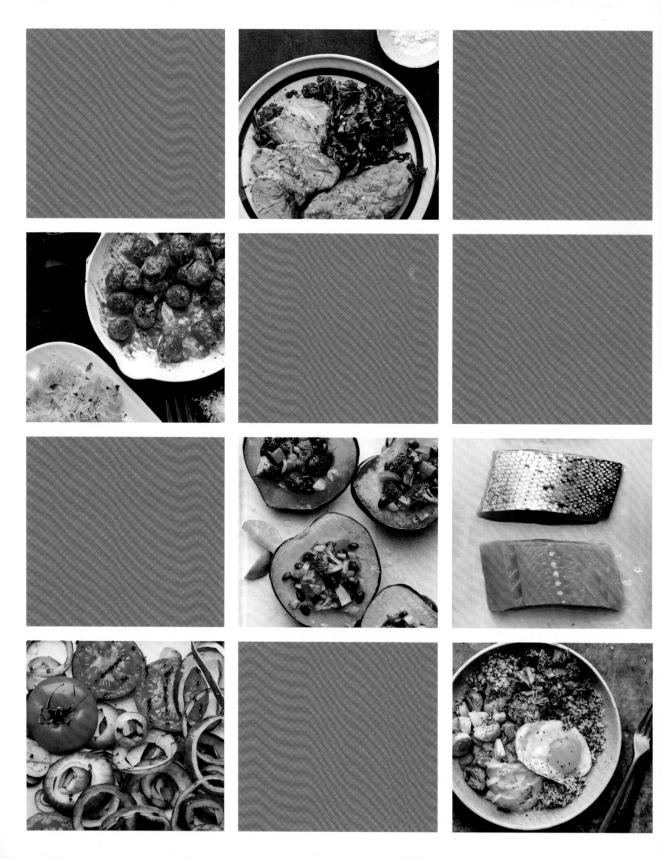

DINNER

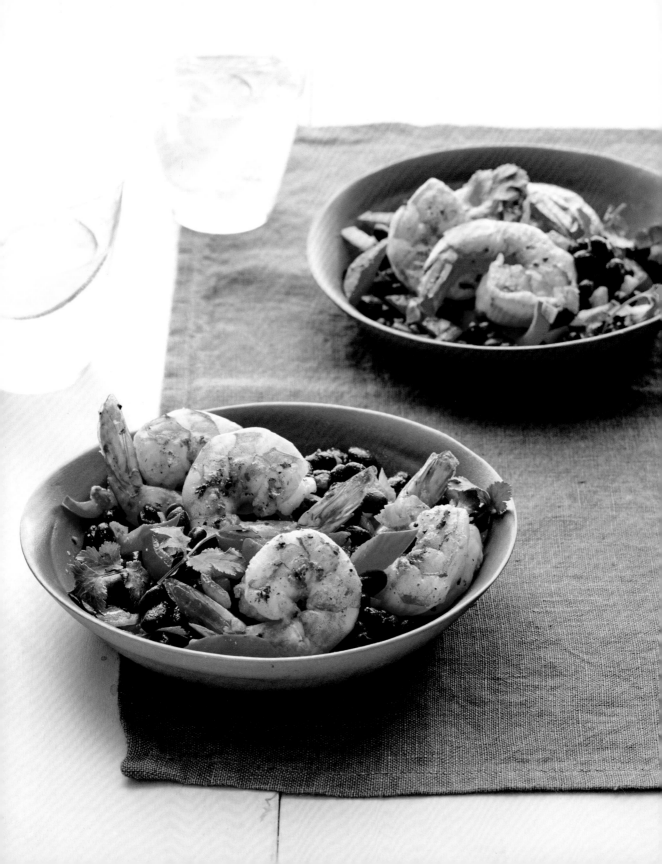

SAUTÉED SHRIMP
ON A WARM BLACK BEAN SALAD

SERVES 6

PER SERVING

CALORIES: 233.3
FAT: 5.1 g
SODIUM: 321.5 mg
CARBOHYDRATE: 21.1 g
FIBER: 7 g
SUGARS: 0.2 g
PROTEIN: 25.8 g

Shrimp used to get a bad rap because of its cholesterol content, but these days dietary cholesterol isn't considered as bad as it once was. That's good news, because shrimp is a great source of lean protein—3 ounces provide about 20 grams of protein with very little fat. It's also low in mercury and provides two helpful antioxidants—selenium and astaxanthin—which may help stave off aging, disease, and inflammation.

IN A MEDIUM NONSTICK SAUTÉ PAN or skillet set over medium heat, heat 2 teaspoons of the oil. Add the onion and bell pepper. Cook, stirring, until soft, about 5 minutes. Stir in the cumin and cook until fragrant, 1 minute. Add the black beans, lime juice, ¼ teaspoon of the salt, and ¼ teaspoon of the black pepper. Cook until heated through, about 3 minutes. Stir in the lime zest. Divide the mixture among 6 serving plates or transfer to a serving platter. Cover to keep warm.

SEASON THE SHRIMP with the remaining ¼ teaspoon salt and ¼ teaspoon black pepper. In the same pan set over medium heat, heat the remaining 2 teaspoons oil. Add the shrimp and cook, stirring, until opaque, about 5 minutes. Divide the shrimp over the bean mixture, sprinkle with cilantro, and serve.

TIP: If choosing between fresh or frozen shrimp, go for frozen! Most commercially caught shrimp are frozen, so what you're seeing at the seafood counter has most likely been thawed. Since you have no idea how long the shrimp has been sitting there, it's best to get frozen and thaw it yourself. To quickly thaw, place in a bowl in a sink and cover with cool water. Change the water every 5 minutes or until the shrimp are soft and flexible.

4 teaspoons olive oil

1 small onion, chopped

1 medium red bell pepper, chopped

1 teaspoon ground cumin

1 (15-ounce) can black beans, rinsed and drained

2 teaspoons fresh lime juice

½ teaspoon coarse salt

½ teaspoon freshly ground black pepper

1 teaspoon grated lime zest

1¼ pounds medium or large shrimp, shelled and deveined (see Tip)

2 tablespoons chopped fresh cilantro leaves

WHOLE ROASTED
STRIPED BASS
WITH CITRUS AND LEEKS
SERVES 2

2 medium leeks (white parts only), cut into thin strips

2 (1½-pound) whole striped bass, cleaned and gutted

4 teaspoons olive oil

¾ teaspoon coarse salt

¾ teaspoon freshly ground black pepper

1 small navel orange, sliced

1 lemon, sliced

½ bunch fresh thyme

Fish is definitely an athlete's ally. Besides its high protein content, fish is low in saturated fat and a great source of minerals like calcium, phosphorus, magnesium, iron, and zinc. One of the easiest ways to cook fish is to roast it whole. All you have to do is buy it cleaned and gutted, then stuff the inside cavity with aromatics and bake it. Serve with a salad or vegetables, such as Balsamic Mushrooms (page 207), and you have a great meal.

PREHEAT THE OVEN to 425°F. Line a rimmed baking sheet big enough to accommodate both fish with parchment paper.

PLACE TWO MOUNDS of leeks on the prepared baking sheet and arrange the fish on top. Rub the insides of each with 1 teaspoon of the oil, ¼ teaspoon of the salt, and ¼ teaspoon of the pepper. Stuff the cavities with the orange and lemon slices and the thyme. Close the cavities and firmly pat down to enclose the citrus and thyme. Rub the remaining 2 teaspoons oil on top of each. Season with the remaining ½ teaspoon salt and ½ teaspoon pepper.

ROAST until the fish is cooked through, 15 to 20 minutes. Serve immediately.

POACHED SALMON SALAD
WITH DILL-CAPER SAUCE
SERVES 4

PER SERVING

CALORIES: 272.4
FAT: 11.1 g
SODIUM: 960 mg
CARBOHYDRATE: 3.1 g
FIBER: 0.8 g
SUGARS: 1.8 g
PROTEIN: 37.1 g

Salmon is a terrific food that I highly recommend to all my clients. Not only is it a source of high-quality protein, but it's also rich in omega-3 fatty acids. Found in other fish like tuna, mackerel, and sardines, and some plants, omega-3s may reduce the risk of heart disease, chronic disease, and inflammation (key for the athlete). They've also been shown in some studies to benefit the brain. In this recipe, we use the technique of poaching to cook the salmon. Not only is it a gentle way of cooking the fish, but it also keeps the salmon moist without adding any fat.

- 1½ teaspoons salt
- 2 tablespoons plus 1 teaspoon fresh lemon juice
- 1½ teaspoons white wine vinegar
- 4 salmon fillets (6 ounces each)
- ½ cup plain nonfat Greek yogurt, such as Fage
- 1 teaspoon mayonnaise
- ¼ teaspoon Dijon mustard
- 2 teaspoons capers, drained
- 1½ teaspoons chopped fresh dill
- ¼ teaspoon grated lemon zest
- ¼ teaspoon coarse salt
- Pinch of freshly ground black pepper
- 1 (5-ounce) bag mixed field greens (see Tip)

IN A LARGE, DEEP SAUTÉ PAN set over high heat, bring 1 quart of water, the salt, 2 tablespoons of the lemon juice, and the vinegar to a boil. Gently place the salmon fillets in a single layer in the pan. If the water level is too low, add enough to just cover the fish. Turn the heat down to low so that the liquid barely simmers. Poach the fish until it flakes easily with a fork, about 10 minutes. Transfer the fish to a plate and let cool.

IN A SMALL BOWL, whisk together the yogurt, mayonnaise, mustard, capers, dill, lemon zest, salt, and pepper.

DIVIDE THE GREENS among 4 serving plates. Top with the warm fish and spoon the sauce over the fish.

TIP: Not in the mood for salad? Omit the greens and serve the salmon and sauce with a side of steamed veggies like broccoli or green beans.

CITRUS-SOY
GLAZED SALMON
WITH BABY BOK CHOY

SERVES 4

¼ cup honey

3 tablespoons low-sodium soy sauce

2 tablespoons sesame oil

2 tablespoons fresh lemon juice

2 tablespoons rice wine vinegar

1 teaspoon grated ginger

½ teaspoon crushed red pepper flakes (optional)

4 salmon fillets (6 ounces each)

8 heads baby bok choy (see Tip, opposite)

1 tablespoon olive or canola oil

1 teaspoon toasted sesame seeds

Fuel up on this Asian-inspired dish that features omega-3-rich salmon. Briefly marinating the fish and basting during cooking allow the salmon to absorb the bright and flavorful marinade that features lemon juice and grated ginger. This dish is great with a side of quinoa. As we know, consuming omega-3s should always be a priority for the athlete, and this dish is a tasty way to accomplish that goal.

IN A MEDIUM BOWL, whisk together the honey, soy sauce, sesame oil, lemon juice, vinegar, ginger, and red pepper flakes (if using).

PREHEAT THE OVEN to 400°F.

PLACE THE SALMON FILLETS in a baking dish skin side down, and pour half of the marinade on top. Let sit, turning several times, for 10 to 15 minutes.

BAKE, basting with the marinade every 5 minutes or so, until the fish is opaque, 15 to 20 minutes.

MEANWHILE, slice the bok choy in half, or if very large, into quarters. In a large nonstick skillet set over medium-high heat, heat the olive oil. When the oil begins to shimmer, add the bok choy and cook, turning several times, until browned and the leaves are wilted, 3 to 4 minutes. Turn off the heat and pour just enough of the remaining marinade on top of the bok choy to coat it.

TRANSFER THE BOK CHOY to a serving platter and top with the salmon fillets. Sprinkle toasted sesame seeds on top, and serve hot.

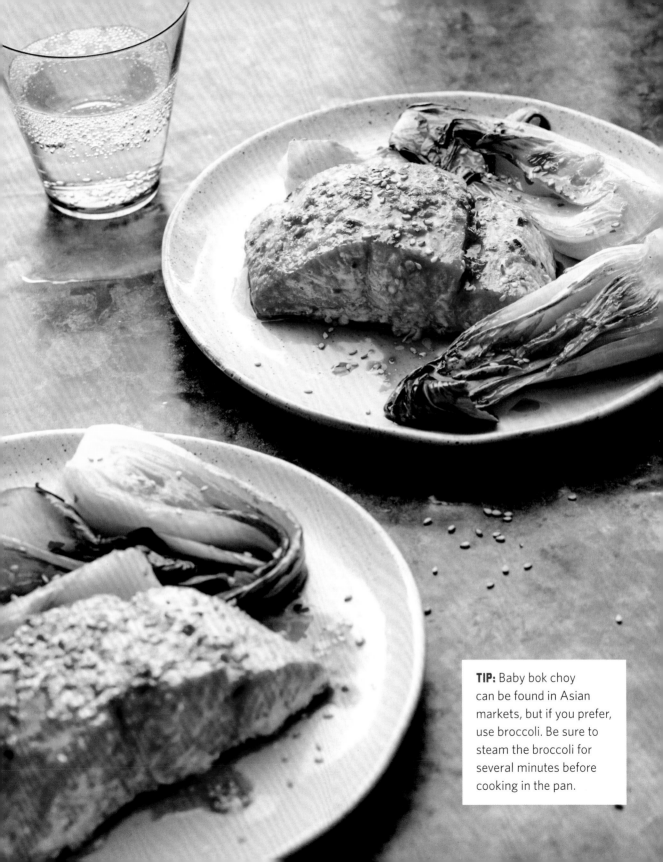

TIP: Baby bok choy can be found in Asian markets, but if you prefer, use broccoli. Be sure to steam the broccoli for several minutes before cooking in the pan.

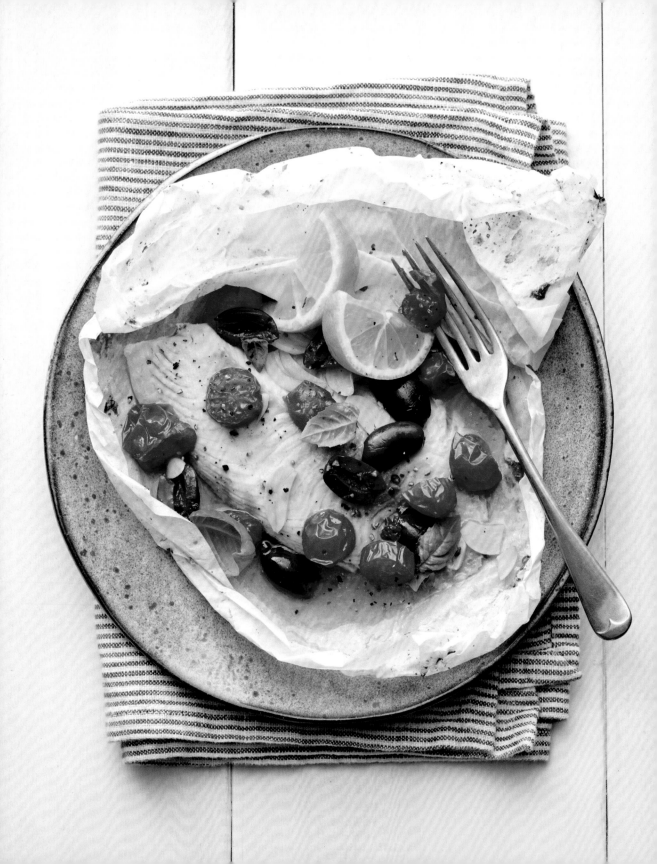

PARCHMENT-BAKED
TILAPIA
WITH TOMATO, BASIL, AND GARLIC

SERVES 4

PER SERVING

CALORIES: 271.4
FAT: 12.3 g
SODIUM: 951.9 mg
CARBOHYDRATE: 7.8 g
FIBER: 1.7 g
SUGARS: 0 g
PROTEIN: 34.7 g

Cooking food in parchment is a classic, healthy technique that yields flavorful results. Foods like vegetables, fish, and poultry steam in their juices, allowing them to stay moist and maintain their own flavor without the need for much added fat. The idea of baking food in parchment paper may seem fussy, but it's actually easier than you think. If you don't have parchment on hand, you can use aluminum foil.

- 4 tilapia fillets (6 ounces each)
- 4 ounces cherry or grape tomatoes
- 12 pitted kalamata olives, roughly chopped
- 4 small garlic cloves, thinly sliced
- 20 fresh basil leaves
- 1 teaspoon coarse salt
- ½ teaspoon freshly ground black pepper
- 4 teaspoons extra-virgin olive oil
- 1 lemon, cut into 4 wedges

PREHEAT THE OVEN to 400°F. Fold four 12 × 14-inch pieces of parchment paper in half. Using scissors, cut the paper into half heart shapes. Unfold the papers.

PLACE EACH FILLET on one side of a piece of paper. Equally divide the tomatoes, olives, garlic, and basil among the fillets. Season with salt and pepper. Drizzle the oil and squeeze a wedge of lemon over each fillet. Fold the parchment over and, starting from one of the ends, fold and crimp the edges to tightly seal. Repeat with the other fillets. Place the packets on rimmed baking sheets.

BAKE until the fish is firm, 15 to 20 minutes. Serve immediately, with or without the parchment packet.

TURKEY CUTLETS
WITH SPINACH, PEARS, AND BLUE CHEESE

SERVES 4

- 1 teaspoon dried sage
- 1 teaspoon dried thyme
- 1 teaspoon dried marjoram
- ¾ teaspoon coarse salt
- ¼ teaspoon plus ⅛ teaspoon freshly ground black pepper
- 4 extra lean turkey cutlets (about 4 ounces each)
- Canola oil cooking spray
- 1 (12-ounce) package (or bunch) of fresh spinach
- 1 tablespoon light butter (see Tip, page 103)
- 1 firm medium pear, cored and thinly sliced
- ¼ cup crumbled blue cheese, for serving

This sweet-and-savory dinner gives you all you need for a solid core diet meal: protein, fat, and carbs (not to mention a healthy dose of both fruit and vegetables!). This versatile dish can also be transformed into a lunch salad by leaving the spinach raw and topping the greens with the turkey and pears. I'm getting hungry just thinking about it!

IN A SMALL BOWL, combine the sage, thyme, marjoram, ½ teaspoon of the salt, and ¼ teaspoon of the pepper. Rub the mixture all over the turkey cutlets.

SPRAY A LARGE NONSTICK SKILLET or sauté pan with cooking spray and set it over medium heat. Add the cutlets and cook until browned on one side, 4 to 5 minutes. Flip the cutlets and cook until cooked through, 4 to 5 minutes. Transfer to a plate and cover with foil to keep warm.

IN THE SAME PAN over medium heat, spray with a little more cooking spray and cook the spinach, stirring, until just wilted, about 3 minutes. Season with the remaining ¼ teaspoon salt and ⅛ teaspoon pepper. Transfer the spinach to a serving platter.

IN THE SAME PAN over medium heat, melt the butter. Add the pear slices and cook, stirring occasionally, until tender and lightly browned, about 5 minutes.

TO SERVE, top the spinach with the turkey and pear slices. Sprinkle with the blue cheese.

TURKEY-MOZZARELLA
MEAT LOAF

SERVES 4

This recipe is a favorite among my clients. I love beef-based meat loaf as much as the next person, but it can be extremely heavy and limit the next workout, never mind being loaded with fat. Here, I lightened up the average meat loaf and came up with this nutritious version that features lean ground turkey and vitamin- and mineral-packed spinach. For a little decadence, I added a layer of mozzarella cheese for flavor and a dose of bone-building calcium. It's incredibly easy to make and keeps in the fridge all week long for quick lunches and dinners.

PREHEAT THE OVEN to 375°F. Generously coat the inside of an 8½ × 4½-inch loaf pan with cooking spray.

IN A LARGE BOWL, combine the turkey, spinach, onion, bread crumbs, parsley, oregano, egg whites, salt, and pepper. Using a spatula, gently mix together until just combined. Press half of the mixture into the bottom of the prepared pan. Scatter an even layer of the cheese on top, and then cover with the remaining turkey mixture. Smooth the top.

BAKE until an instant-read thermometer inserted into the loaf registers 160°F., about 35 minutes. Let cool slightly before slicing and serving.

TIP: Ground turkey can sometimes be made with dark meat or a combination of dark and white meat, which makes it fattier than lean ground meat. Be sure to look for ground turkey that's labeled "lean" on the package or contains less than 10% fat.

Canola oil cooking spray
1½ pounds 93% lean ground turkey (see Tip)
1 (10-ounce) package of frozen chopped spinach, thawed and excess water removed
½ cup chopped onion
½ cup seasoned dry bread crumbs
¼ cup chopped fresh flat-leaf parsley
1 teaspoon dried oregano
2 large egg whites
½ teaspoon coarse salt
¼ teaspoon freshly ground black pepper
4 ounces grated part-skim mozzarella cheese

PER SERVING

CALORIES: 274.2
FAT: 15.8 g
SODIUM: 215.9 mg
CARBOHYDRATE: 24.5 g
FIBER: 6.3 g
SUGARS: 12.1 g
PROTEIN: 12.3 g

ORANGE AND FENNEL SALAD
WITH SHREDDED CHICKEN
SERVES 4

- 3 medium navel oranges
- 2 tablespoons white wine vinegar
- 2 tablespoons fresh orange juice
- 1½ teaspoons honey
- ½ small shallot, chopped
- ¼ cup extra-virgin olive oil
- ¼ teaspoon coarse salt
- ¼ teaspoon freshly ground black pepper
- 2½ ounces field greens
- 2 medium fennel bulbs, thinly sliced
- 1 cup shredded rotisserie chicken breast

Fennel is a good source of vitamin C, potassium, and fiber, and it's delicious either cooked or eaten raw, as in this salad. Use a sharp knife or a mandoline to shave off paper-thin slices—and be very careful!

USING A ZESTER or rasplike tool, remove about 1 teaspoon of zest from the oranges while avoiding the bitter white pith; set aside. Cut off ¼ inch from the top and bottom of the fruit. Using a sharp paring knife, cut the peel away from the orange, following the contours of the fruit. While holding an orange in one hand, cut between the membranes to remove the segments, dropping them into a medium bowl. Squeeze the juices from the membranes into the bowl, reserving 2 tablespoons for the vinaigrette.

IN A SEPARATE MEDIUM BOWL, whisk together the vinegar, reserved orange juice and zest, honey, and shallot. In a steady stream, pour in the oil while whisking. Season with the salt and pepper.

IN A LARGE BOWL, toss together the greens, fennel, and three quarters of the dressing. Arrange the orange sections and chicken on top, and drizzle with the remaining dressing. Serve immediately.

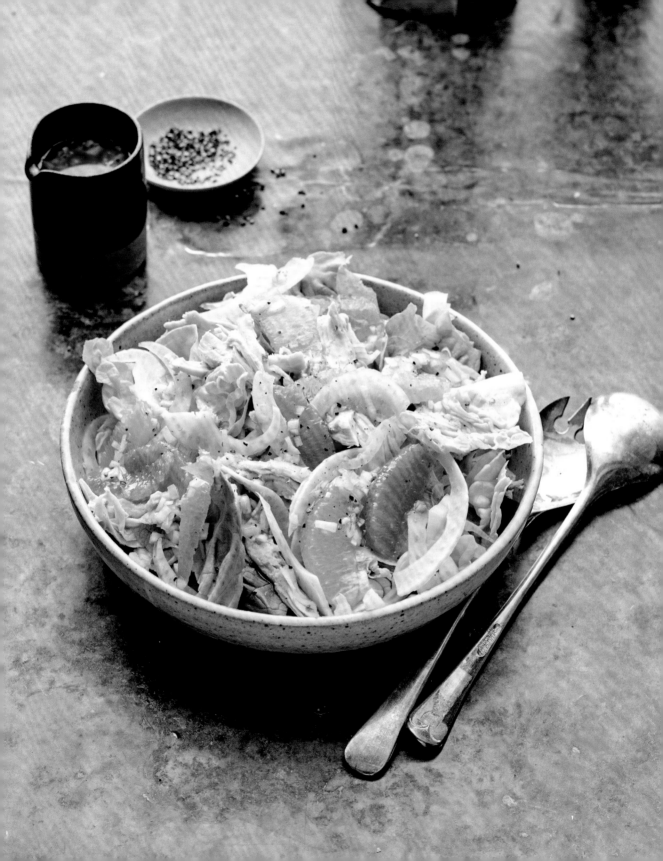

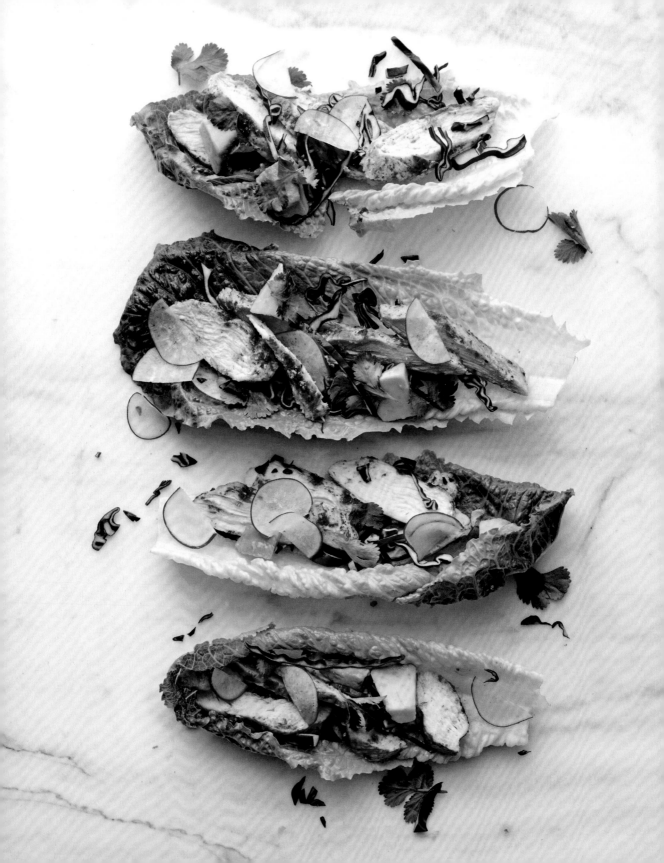

CHIPOTLE CHICKEN TACOS

MAKES 12 TACOS: SERVES 4

PER SERVING

CALORIES: 340.3
FAT: 15.4 g
SODIUM: 1,225.7 mg
CARBOHYDRATE: 11 g
FIBER: 6 g
SUGARS: 2.1 g
PROTEIN: 41 g

You may think that tacos are off the table with the core diet, but think again. Here, we replaced grain-based tortillas with lettuce leaves, which are low in calories and have a great crunchy texture. Try firm lettuces like romaine and butter lettuce, because they can stand up to the weight of the filling. As a variation, you can also use a product such as Joseph's brand Flax, Oat Bran & Whole Wheat Flour Tortillas in place of the lettuce to make a burrito!

PLACE THE CHICKEN BREASTS between sheets of waxed paper. Using a meat mallet or heavy skillet, pound the breasts until they are about ½ to ¾ inch thick.

IN A SMALL BOWL, combine the chili powder, salt, garlic powder, and onion powder. Sprinkle the mixture all over the chicken, and then rub 2 teaspoons of the oil on the chicken.

HEAT A GRILL PAN over medium-high heat. Using tongs, rub the grates of the pan with an oil-soaked paper towel. Place the chicken on the grill and cook until cooked through, about 5 minutes per side. Transfer to a cutting board and cut crosswise into ½-inch-thick strips.

SERVE THE CHICKEN in the lettuce leaves topped with the avocado, sliced radishes, shredded red cabbage, and cilantro. Serve lime wedges on the side.

1½ pounds boneless, skinless chicken breast
2 tablespoons chipotle chili powder
2 teaspoons coarse salt
1 teaspoon garlic powder
1 teaspoon onion powder
2 teaspoons canola oil, plus more for the pan
12 medium romaine or butter lettuce leaves
1 medium avocado, pitted and chopped
3 medium radishes, thinly sliced
2 cups shredded red cabbage
¼ cup chopped fresh cilantro leaves
1 lime, cut into wedges

PER SERVING

CALORIES: 261.1
FAT: 16.9 g
SODIUM: 586 mg
CARBOHYDRATE: 11.3 g
FIBER: 1.3 g
SUGARS: 6.5 g
PROTEIN: 17.8 g

CHICKEN MEATBALLS
OVER SPAGHETTI SQUASH

SERVES 6

1 small to medium spaghetti squash (about 1 pound)

3 tablespoons olive oil

1 pound 93% lean ground chicken

1 small onion, finely chopped

1 small garlic clove, finely chopped

¼ cup grated Parmesan cheese, plus more for serving (optional)

1 large egg

2 tablespoons chopped parsley, plus more for serving

2 tablespoons chopped basil, plus more for serving

½ teaspoon coarse salt

¼ teaspoon freshly ground black pepper

1¼ cups no-sugar-added marinara sauce

This version of traditional spaghetti and meatballs features chicken rather than beef. To keep the meatballs from being too dry and firm, I use 93% lean ground chicken, which can be found in most supermarkets, and make them bite-size, so they don't take too long to cook. For those of you looking to keep your iron up, feel free to use ground beef instead, though it isn't as lean as the chicken used here.

PREHEAT THE OVEN to 400°F.

USING A SHARP KNIFE, carefully slice the squash in half lengthwise. Remove the seeds and discard. Rub 1 tablespoon of the oil over the squash and place cut side down on a baking sheet. Roast until a knife can be easily inserted into the squash, 30 to 45 minutes. Let cool.

MEANWHILE, in a medium bowl, combine the chicken, onion, garlic, ¼ cup Parmesan, egg, parsley, basil, salt, and pepper. Using a 1-tablespoon scoop or your hands, form the mixture into small meatballs (see Tip, opposite).

IN A LARGE NONSTICK SKILLET set over medium heat, heat the remaining 2 tablespoons oil. Working in batches, cook the meatballs until browned on all sides, about 10 minutes. Transfer to a plate.

IN THE SAME PAN, heat the marinara sauce until bubbly. Return the meatballs to the pan and simmer for 5 minutes.

USING A FORK, scrape the insides of the spaghetti squash and pile the spaghetti-like noodles onto a serving platter. Top with the meatballs and sauce. Sprinkle Parmesan (if using) and herbs on top, and serve.

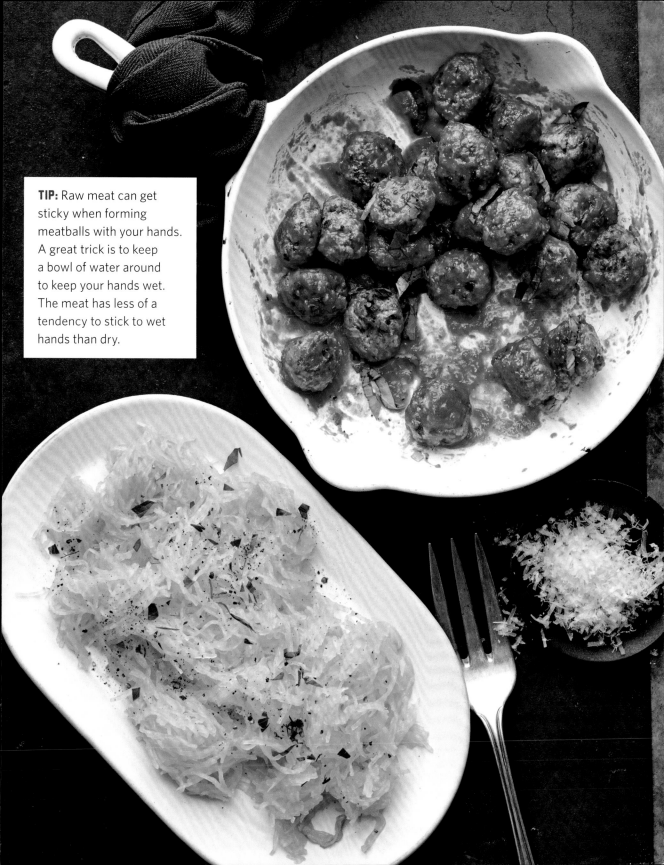

TIP: Raw meat can get sticky when forming meatballs with your hands. A great trick is to keep a bowl of water around to keep your hands wet. The meat has less of a tendency to stick to wet hands than dry.

PER SERVING

CALORIES: 296.3
FAT: 13 g
SODIUM: 358.2 mg
CARBOHYDRATE: 23.2 g
FIBER: 6 g
SUGARS: 5.7 g
PROTEIN: 23.4 g

ASIAN CHICKEN SALAD

SERVES 4

1½ pounds cabbage, shredded (see Tip)
1 cup shredded carrot
1 medium red bell pepper, cored, seeded, and thinly sliced
1 cup shelled edamame
6 radishes, thinly sliced
1½ cups shredded rotisserie chicken breast
1 medium scallion (white and green parts), chopped
2 tablespoons canola oil
2 tablespoons toasted sesame oil
2 tablespoons rice vinegar
4 teaspoons honey
2½ teaspoons low-sodium soy sauce
2 teaspoons finely grated fresh ginger
2 teaspoons toasted sesame seeds (see Tip, page 99)

Asian-inspired chicken salads are usually topped with chow mein noodles or fried wonton strips, both of which are pretty devoid of nutrient density and raise blood sugar quickly. But this core-ratio-friendly, quick-and-easy version features lots of crispy, colorful vegetables that are nutritious and replicate the crunch of those toppings without all the empty, high-glycemic carbs. I also add a good helping of filling protein in this salad to keep hunger at bay.

IN THE BOTTOM of a large serving bowl or platter, arrange the shredded cabbage. Scatter the carrot, bell pepper, edamame, radishes, chicken, and scallion on top.

IN A SMALL BOWL, whisk together the canola oil, sesame oil, vinegar, honey, soy sauce, ginger, and sesame seeds. Drizzle the dressing over the salad and serve.

TIP: In a pinch? Use bagged coleslaw mix in place of the cabbage and carrots. You can find it near the packaged greens in the produce section of your supermarket.

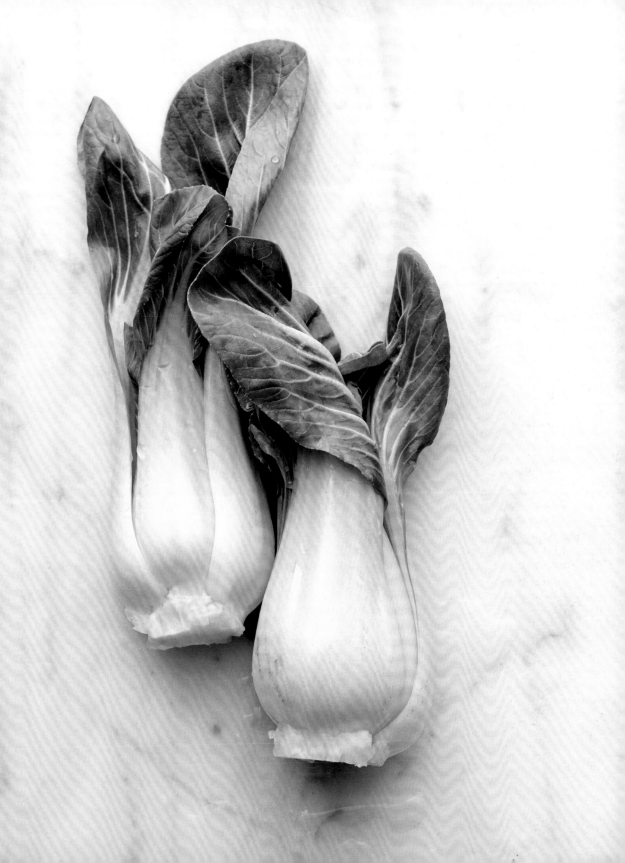

BUTTERNUT SQUASH,
SWEET POTATO, AND APPLE SOUP

MAKES ABOUT 8 CUPS: SERVES 4

- 1 tablespoon extra-virgin olive oil
- 1 tablespoon light butter (see Tip, page 103)
- 1 large Vidalia onion, chopped
- 2 teaspoons dried thyme
- 1 large butternut squash, peeled, seeded, and chopped (about 2¼ pounds)
- 1 medium sweet potato, peeled and chopped (about 10 ounces)
- 1 medium apple, peeled, cored, and chopped
- 3½ cups hot vegetable broth (28 ounces)
- ¼ cup half-and-half (optional)

Rich and creamy, this soup takes advantage of the fall bounty of vegetables. Thanks to the butternut squash and sweet potato, you'll get a hefty dose of beta-carotene, a pigment that gives the vegetables their vibrant red-orange color and protects the body from oxidative damage. Beta-carotene is also converted by the body into vitamin A, which can help maintain a healthy immune system. Have your recovery drink immediately postworkout, and then 1 to 3 hours later, dive into this soup! After the toughest days of training, combining this with Slow-Cooker Turkey Chili (page 135) makes a hearty, filling meal!

IN A LARGE SAUCEPAN set over medium-high heat, heat the oil and butter. When the oil begins to shimmer, add the onion. Cook, stirring, until soft, 2 to 3 minutes. Add the thyme and cook for 1 more minute. Add the squash, sweet potato, and apple, and cook, stirring constantly, for 10 minutes. Pour the vegetable broth into the pan. Cover and bring to a boil. Reduce the heat to low, cover, and simmer until the vegetables are very soft, 20 to 30 minutes. Using an immersion blender (or working in batches with a regular blender), puree the soup until smooth. Stir in the half-and-half (if using). If the soup is too thin, cook over medium heat until the desired consistency is reached. Serve hot.

PORK TENDERLOIN
WITH SWEET POTATOES AND KALE

SERVES 4

PER SERVING

CALORIES: 444.8
FAT: 20.8 g
SODIUM: 778.5 mg
CARBOHYDRATE: 20.9 g
FIBER: 3.3 g
SUGARS: 0.9 g
PROTEIN: 42.5 g

Pork can sometimes get fatty, and therefore high in cholesterol and saturated fat. But some cuts of pork, such as tenderloin, can be just as lean as chicken breast. In fact, a 3-ounce portion of pork tenderloin comes in at 93 calories and 2 grams of fat (0.5 gram of saturated fat). The same amount of boneless, skinless chicken breast clocks in at 102 calories and 2 grams of fat (0.5 gram of saturated fat). In this recipe, I roast a pork tenderloin with garlic and herbs, which give this lean protein excellent flavor.

- 2 medium sweet potatoes (about 1½ pounds)
- 6 garlic cloves
- ¼ teaspoon dried thyme
- ¼ teaspoon dried sage
- 1¼ teaspoons coarse salt
- 4 tablespoons olive oil
- 1 to 1¼ pounds pork tenderloin, silverskin removed
- Bunch of kale, stems removed, chopped

PREHEAT THE OVEN to 450°F.

WASH AND SCRUB the sweet potatoes, prick with a fork, and wrap in foil. Roast until soft and tender, about 45 minutes. Let cool.

MEANWHILE, in a mini food processor or mortar and pestle, combine 4 of the garlic cloves, the thyme, sage, 1 teaspoon of the salt, and 2 tablespoons of the oil. Blend or work the mixture together until it resembles a paste.

PLACE THE TENDERLOIN in a roasting pan and rub the garlic paste all over it. Roast for 10 to 15 minutes. Turn the tenderloin over and roast until an instant-read thermometer inserted into the thickest part of the meat registers 155°F., about 10 more minutes. Transfer the pork to a cutting board and tent with foil. Let sit for 5 minutes before slicing. Cut into 2-inch-thick slices to serve.

recipe continues

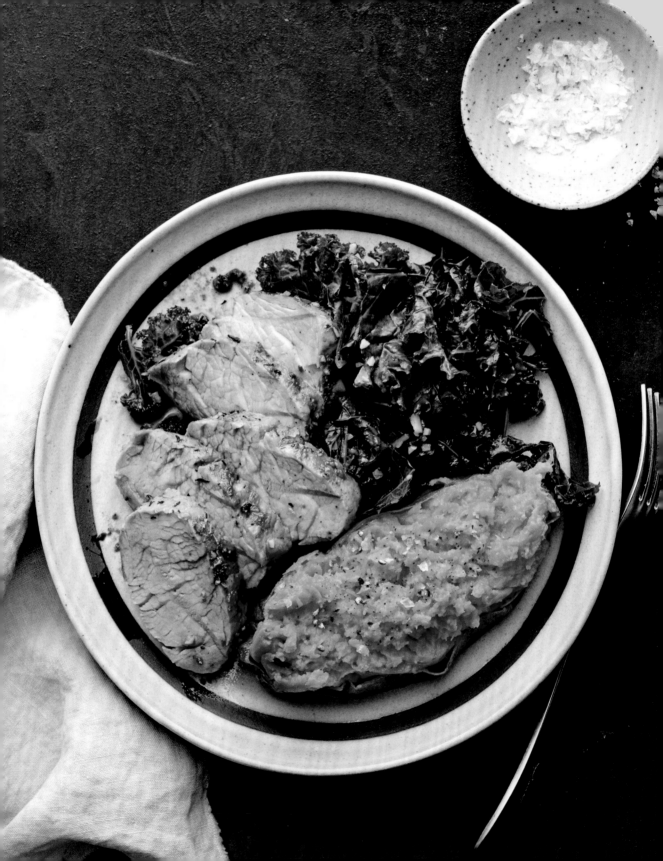

IN A LARGE SAUTÉ PAN or skillet set over medium-high heat, heat the remaining 2 tablespoons oil. Slice the remaining 2 garlic cloves, add them to the pan, and cook for 1 minute. Add the kale and cook until just wilted, 2 minutes. Season with the remaining ¼ teaspoon salt.

UNWRAP THE POTATOES and cut them in half lengthwise. Using your fingers, push the ends of the potatoes so that the flesh pops out. Place each half on a plate. Divide the pork slices and sautéed kale among the plates, and serve.

TIP: Sweet potatoes are carbohydrate-packed root vegetables that also have lots of dietary fiber and beta-carotene. For endurance athletes, they're excellent, convenient, and reliable sources of fuel—and they also happen to be delicious. They're easy to roast, as we do in this recipe, and can be enjoyed many other ways, too. Try making the Sweet Potato Hash with Eggs (page 108), Baked Sweet Potato Chips (page 156), or Butternut Squash, Sweet Potato, and Apple Soup (page 178). And did you know that there are many varieties of sweet potatoes, in colors ranging from white to purple? There's a whole rainbow of options, and each one is a tasty, healthy perfect source of the carbohydrates an endurance athlete needs.

PER SERVING

CALORIES: 395.1
FAT: 26.5 g
SODIUM: 827.7 mg
CARBOHYDRATE: 8 g
FIBER: 2 g
SUGARS: 0.1 g
PROTEIN: 33.6 g

STRIP STEAK
WITH PARSLEY-GARLIC SAUCE
SERVES 4

1 cup packed fresh flat-leaf parsley

2 garlic cloves

½ teaspoon dried oregano

3 tablespoons extra-virgin olive oil

2 tablespoons red wine vinegar

1½ teaspoons coarse salt

1 medium yellow or red onion, sliced crosswise

2 beefsteak tomatoes, sliced in half crosswise

1 tablespoon canola or vegetable oil, plus more for brushing

¾ to 1 pound lean steak, such as strip (top loin), at room temperature (see Tip)

Depending on the cut, steak can be a core-friendly food. In fact, we generally recommend that endurance athletes eat red meat once a week to support healthy iron levels. Fat, saturated fat, and cholesterol content is highly dependent on what part of the animal the meat comes from, and in this recipe, I chose strip steak for its flavor, relative leanness, and suitability for grilling. While there are even leaner cuts of beef, they may not be ideal for grilling as they can be quite tough.

IN A FOOD PROCESSOR OR BLENDER, combine the parsley, garlic, oregano, olive oil, vinegar, and 1 teaspoon of the salt. Blend until pureed.

HEAT A GRILL PAN over high heat. Brush the onion slices and tomato halves with canola oil. Grill until grill marks appear, 2 to 3 minutes per side. Transfer to a plate and tent with foil to keep warm. Scrape any food bits off of the grates when finished.

RUB 1 TABLESPOON of the canola oil on the steak and season with the remaining ½ teaspoon salt. Grill for 6 to 8 minutes total for medium-rare, or until desired doneness.

SLICE THE STEAKS into strips and serve with the onion, tomatoes, and sauce on the side.

TIP: Cuts of meat marked as "lean" must contain less than 10 grams of total fat, 4.5 grams of saturated fat, and 95 milligrams of cholesterol per 3½-ounce serving. "Extra lean" must have less than 5 grams of total fat, 2 grams of saturated fat, and 95 milligrams of cholesterol. For the purposes of the core diet, "lean" is sufficient to avoid significant amounts of saturated fat, which has been linked to heart disease.

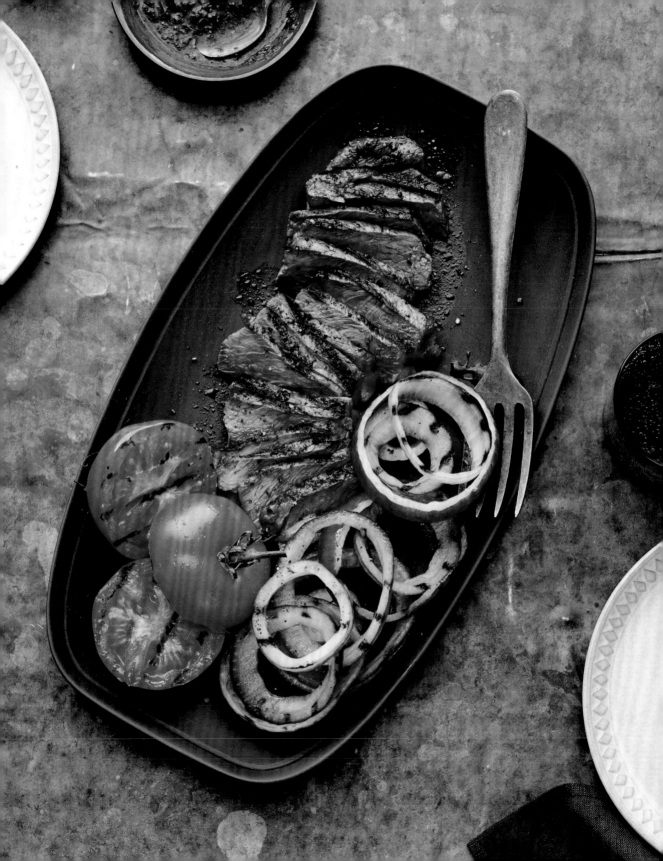

BEEF AND QUINOA
STUFFED PEPPERS
SERVES 6

½ cup quinoa
3 medium green or red bell peppers (see Tip, opposite)
1 tablespoon olive oil
½ medium yellow onion, chopped
1 garlic clove, chopped
1½ teaspoons sodium-free Italian seasoning
8 ounces 90% lean ground beef
1¼ cups no-sugar-added marinara sauce
½ cup grated carrot
½ teaspoon coarse salt
¼ teaspoon freshly ground black pepper
3 tablespoons grated Parmesan cheese

Try this protein- and veggie-packed meal when you want something satisfying, but not too heavy. This dish is similar to traditional stuffed peppers, but we swapped saturated-fat-laden ground chuck with 90% lean ground beef. And to keep the meat flavorful and moist, we added aromatics like onion and garlic, along with quinoa and grated carrot. Try including other leftover veggies if you'd like.

PREHEAT THE OVEN to 400°F.

COOK THE QUINOA according to the package directions.

SLICE THE BELL PEPPERS in half lengthwise and remove the core and seeds. Place them cut side up in a 9 × 13-inch baking dish. Set aside.

IN A LARGE NONSTICK SAUTÉ PAN or skillet set over medium-high heat, heat the oil. When the oil begins to shimmer, add the onion and garlic. Cook, stirring, until soft, 5 minutes. Stir in the Italian seasoning and cook for 1 more minute. Add the beef and cook, using the back of a wooden spoon to break up any lumps, until browned through, 5 to 7 minutes. Add the cooked quinoa, 1 cup of the marinara sauce, the carrot, salt, and black pepper. Spoon the mixture into the cavities of the bell peppers.

IN A SMALL BOWL, combine the remaining ¼ cup marinara sauce with ¾ cup water and pour into the bottom of the baking dish. Tightly cover the dish with foil.

BAKE UNTIL THE BELL PEPPERS are tender, about 30 minutes. Uncover and sprinkle the cheese on top of the bell peppers. Bake until the cheese is melted, 5 more minutes. Spoon the pan juices on top of the bell peppers and serve.

TIP: Vitamin C is a known for helping the body defend against the common cold and as a great antioxidant for endurance athletes. While most people associate oranges with this vitamin, bell peppers actually have higher levels of it. In fact, 1 cup of chopped bell peppers has twice as much vitamin C as 1 cup of orange segments.

PER SERVING

CALORIES: 389.2
FAT: 7.8 g
SODIUM: 1,271.6 mg
CARBOHYDRATE: 61.8 g
FIBER: 20.2 g
SUGARS: 7 g
PROTEIN: 19.8 g

VEGETARIAN
THREE-BEAN CHILI

MAKES 10 CUPS; SERVES 5

2 tablespoons olive oil
1 medium onion, chopped
3 garlic cloves, chopped
2 teaspoons ground cumin
1 teaspoon dried oregano
1 teaspoon chipotle chili powder
1 small zucchini, chopped
1 small yellow squash, chopped
½ medium red bell pepper, chopped
1 (6-ounce) can tomato paste
1 (15.5-ounce) can black beans, rinsed and drained (see Tip)
1 (15.5-ounce) can chickpeas, rinsed and drained
1 (15.5-ounce) can red kidney beans, rinsed and drained
1 (10-ounce) can diced tomatoes with chiles
1 (14.5-ounce) can fire-roasted diced tomatoes
1¼ teaspoons coarse salt

With three different types of hearty, protein-packed beans, lots of colorful veggies, and a spicy kick from chipotle chili powder, this dish is a knockout. Chipotles are smoked and dried jalapeño peppers; when ground, some say they have a spicier flavor than jalapeños. This meal is truly a one-pot wonder that'll keep your body humming!

IN A LARGE SAUCEPAN set over medium-high heat, heat the oil. When the oil begins to shimmer, add the onion and garlic. Cook, stirring, until softened, 3 to 5 minutes. Stir in the cumin, oregano, and chili powder, and cook, stirring, until fragrant, 1 to 2 minutes. Add the zucchini, yellow squash, and bell pepper, and gently stir to coat the vegetables with the spices. Add 2 cups water, the tomato paste, black beans, chickpeas, kidney beans, tomatoes with chilies, fire-roasted tomatoes, and salt. Stir well and bring to a boil. Reduce the heat to medium-low, cover, and simmer for 25 minutes. Uncover and cook until the chili thickens, 5 more minutes. Serve hot.

TIP: Rinsing canned beans can remove up to 40% of the sodium coating the bean. Although sodium is no enemy to the endurance athlete, during cool months when sweat rates are lower, you likely don't need as much sodium from your day-to-day eating (unless you are doing long indoor stationary bike rides or treadmill runs, in which case sweat rates will be high).

PEANUT AND BUTTERNUT
SQUASH STEW

SERVES 6

PER SERVING

CALORIES: 331.2
FAT: 21.6 g
SODIUM: 249.5 mg
CARBOHYDRATE: 29.1 g
FIBER: 7.8 g
SUGARS: 6.4 g
PROTEIN: 9.7 g

Don't balk! Peanuts and peanut butter are commonly used in stews and other savory dishes in many parts of the world. That rich nuttiness combined with the earthiness of squash is delicious, so be sure to give this one a try. The flavorful spices and abundance of filling vegetables make this vegetarian dish extremely satisfying on hard training days in the winter. You can easily add pork or beef as well, which would of course kick the protein content up a notch.

IN A LARGE POT set over medium-high heat, heat the oil. When the oil begins to shimmer, add the onion and garlic. Cook, stirring, until soft, 5 minutes. Add the turmeric, cumin, coriander, and cinnamon, and cook until fragrant, 1 minute. Stir in 1 cup water, the squash, coconut milk, and tomatoes. Bring to a boil, reduce the heat to low, cover, and simmer until the squash is tender, 10 to 15 minutes. Stir in the peanut butter and kale. Cook until the kale is wilted, 1 to 2 minutes.

LADLE THE STEW into six serving bowls. Top with cilantro (see Tip), peanuts, and a lime wedge. Serve.

TIP: The flavor of fresh leafy herbs becomes muted when added too early during cooking. It's best to add to them in the last couple of minutes to preserve their color and taste.

2 tablespoons extra-virgin olive oil
1 medium yellow onion, chopped
3 garlic cloves, chopped
½ teaspoon ground turmeric
½ teaspoon ground cumin
½ teaspoon ground coriander
½ teaspoon ground cinnamon
4 cups peeled and chopped butternut squash
1 (14-ounce) can light coconut milk
1 (14-ounce) can diced tomatoes
½ cup natural peanut butter, such as Naturally More
½ bunch of kale or Swiss chard, chopped
3 tablespoons chopped fresh cilantro leaves
6 tablespoons chopped unsalted peanuts
Lime wedges, for serving

LENTIL–BLACK BEAN
VEGGIE PATTIES

MAKES 6 PATTIES; SERVES 3

- 1½ cups cooked red or brown lentils (see Tip)
- ½ cup canned black beans, rinsed and drained
- ¾ cup cooked quinoa
- ¼ cup finely chopped onion
- ¼ cup shredded carrot
- ½ cup chopped baby spinach
- ½ teaspoon paprika
- ½ teaspoon ground cumin
- ¼ teaspoon onion powder
- 1 teaspoon coarse salt
- 2 large eggs, beaten
- 2 tablespoons olive oil
- 10 to 12 large romaine lettuce leaves

Many of the prepared veggie burgers that you can buy in stores today too often focus on being meat substitutes, besides being high in sodium and not tasting all that great. These patties, on the other hand, don't even try to pretend to be meat! With high-quality plant protein from lentils, black beans, and quinoa, and nutritious vegetables like carrot and spinach, these are super healthy and mighty tasty, too. Serve with a dollop of roasted red pepper sauce (see page 105), or in a core-ratio-friendly grain product such as Joseph's brand Flax, Oat Bran & Whole Wheat Flour Tortillas.

IN A LARGE BOWL, combine the lentils, black beans, quinoa, onion, carrot, spinach, paprika, cumin, onion powder, and salt. Pour in the eggs and stir to combine. Form the mixture into patties and place on a tray lined with wax or parchment paper. Refrigerate for at least 1 hour.

IN A LARGE SAUTÉ PAN set over medium heat, heat the oil. Gently place the patties in the pan and cook until golden brown on one side, about 3 minutes. Carefully flip the patties and cook until the second side is browned, 2 to 3 minutes. (This can be done in batches.) Serve the patties in lettuce leaves.

TIP: To cook lentils, put them in a pot of boiling water. Bring back to a boil, and then simmer until desired consistency is reached, 20 to 30 minutes. Add extra water, if necessary, to keep the lentils covered.

CAULIFLOWER FRIED "RICE"

SERVES 2

PER SERVING

CALORIES: 297.2
FAT: 10.2 g
SODIUM: 1,180.4 mg
CARBOHYDRATE: 28 g
FIBER: 9.4 g
SUGARS: 2.6 g
PROTEIN: 26.6 g

Fried rice is of course off-limits on the core diet, as rice is a grain. However, this version uses cauliflower "rice," which fills up some of the nutritional void! A member of the cabbage family and a cousin to broccoli and kale, cauliflower is now as popular as ever. Thanks to its mild flavor, versatility, and low carbohydrate content, it's used as a substitute for potatoes, rice, and bread. When I tested this recipe on hungry eaters, some couldn't tell that this wasn't made with rice! I've made it with chicken, but you can omit it if you prefer.

IN THE BOWL OF A FOOD PROCESSOR, place about a third of the cauliflower. Pulse several times until the cauliflower resembles small, ricelike pieces. (Be careful not to overprocess.) Transfer to a large bowl, and repeat processing the remaining cauliflower in batches.

SPRAY A WOK or large sauté pan set over medium-high heat with cooking spray. Pour the eggs into the pan and season with a pinch of salt. Using a spatula, quickly cook and scramble the eggs. Transfer to a small bowl.

IN THE SAME PAN set over medium-high heat, heat the olive and sesame oils. Add the ginger, garlic, onion, and scallion whites. Cook, stirring constantly, until fragrant and soft, about 5 minutes. Stir in the edamame, carrots, and chicken (if using), then the cauliflower and soy sauce. Stir well. Cover and cook for about 3 minutes. Uncover and stir in the eggs and scallion greens.

1 medium head cauliflower, roughly chopped
Canola oil cooking spray
2 large eggs, beaten
Pinch of coarse salt
1 teaspoon olive oil
2 teaspoons sesame oil
½ teaspoon minced fresh ginger
3 garlic cloves, minced
½ small onion, chopped
4 scallions (white and green parts separated), thinly sliced
½ cup shelled edamame
¼ cup shredded or diced carrots
½ cup shredded or chopped chicken (optional)
3 tablespoons low-sodium soy sauce

SUNNY-SIDE-UP EGG AND
QUINOA BOWL
WITH ROASTED VEGETABLES

SERVES 4

1 pound green bell
    peppers
¼ cup plus
    2 tablespoons
    olive oil
1 teaspoon salt
1 cup quinoa
2 tablespoons fresh
    lemon juice
1 tablespoon Dijon
    mustard
1½ teaspoons
    chopped shallot
½ garlic clove
Pinch of freshly
    ground black
    pepper
Olive oil cooking
    spray
4 large eggs
1 cup chopped kale or
    baby greens
1 medium ripe
    avocado, pitted
    and diced
¼ cup shredded
    Parmesan cheese

This satisfying and colorful dinner was inspired by the grain bowls that have been popular lately. Use quinoa as the base, top it with a sunny-side-up egg for protein, and then load it up with nutrient-rich vegetables—the recipe calls for green bell peppers, but you can use any kind of vegetable you like. A small hit of Parmesan cheese gives it some nutty richness, and the lemon vinaigrette lends brightness for a vibrant and healthy meal.

PREHEAT THE OVEN to 425°F. On a rimmed baking sheet, toss the peppers with the 2 tablespoons olive oil and ½ teaspoon of the salt. Roast until browned and tender, 15 to 20 minutes.

PREPARE THE QUINOA according to the package directions.

IN A SMALL BOWL, whisk together the lemon juice, mustard, shallot, garlic, ¼ teaspoon of the salt, and pepper. While still whisking, slowly drizzle in the remaining ¼ cup oil.

COAT A MEDIUM NONSTICK FRYING PAN set over medium heat with cooking spray. Crack the eggs into the pan and cook until the whites are set and the yolk still runny, 1 to 2 minutes. Season with the remaining ¼ teaspoon salt.

TO ASSEMBLE, divide the quinoa among four bowls. Divide the roasted vegetables, kale, and avocado among the bowls, and then top each with a fried egg. Sprinkle the Parmesan over the bowls and drizzle with the dressing.

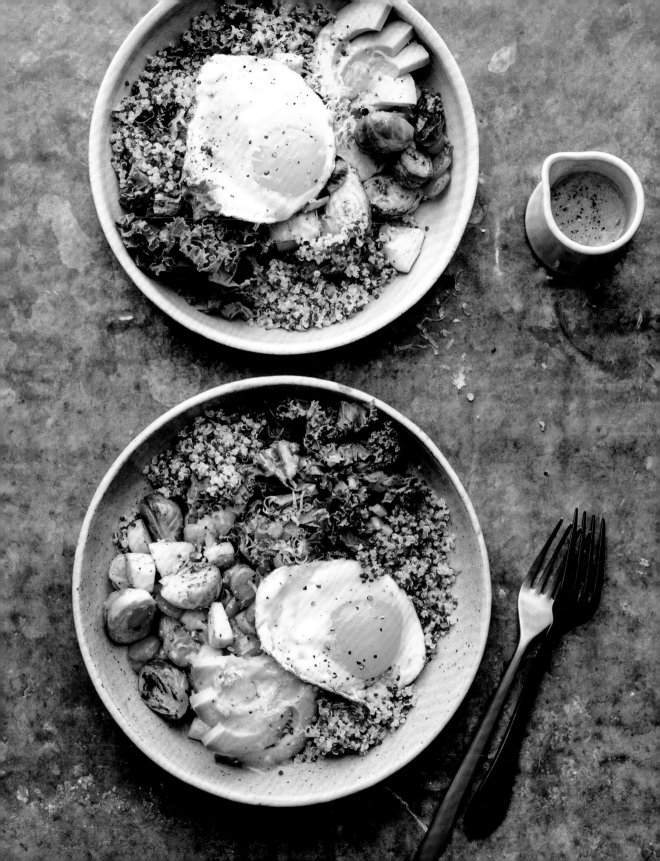

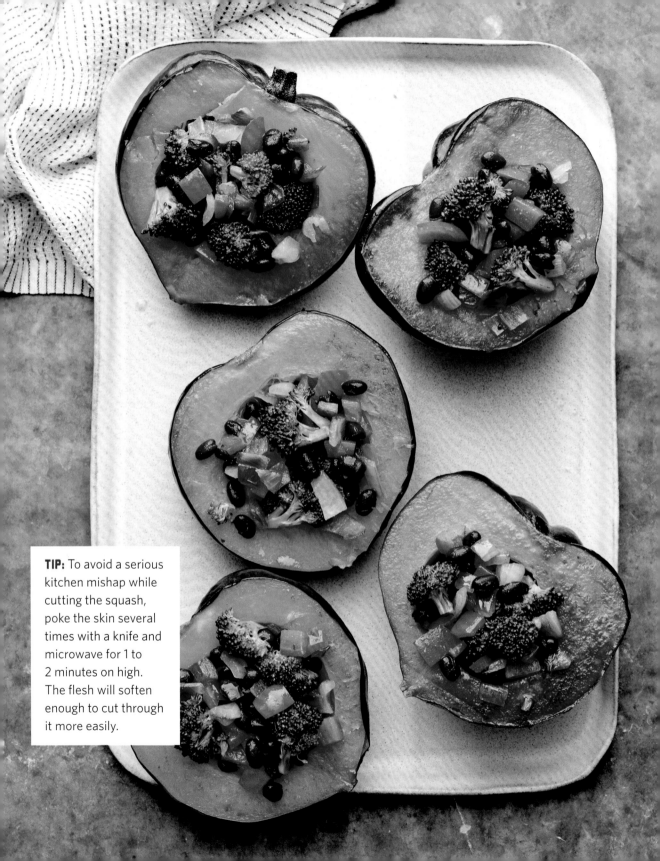

TIP: To avoid a serious kitchen mishap while cutting the squash, poke the skin several times with a knife and microwave for 1 to 2 minutes on high. The flesh will soften enough to cut through it more easily.

SOUTHWESTERN STUFFED
ROASTED ACORN SQUASH

SERVES 6

PER SERVING

CALORIES: 320.4
FAT: 13.2 g
SODIUM: 376.2 mg
CARBOHYDRATE: 46.2 g
FIBER: 11.3 g
SUGARS: 2.8 g
PROTEIN: 9.8 g

Chock-full of nutrients and colors, this vegan dish scores high in satisfaction and flavor. The black beans provide a dose of satiating protein and fiber, along with blood-boosting iron. And the acorn squash, which doubles as a vessel for this dish, provides antioxidants like beta-carotene and vitamin C to help prevent cellular damage from workouts. To save on prep time, I opt for frozen broccoli florets, which are just as nutritious as fresh.

PREHEAT THE OVEN to 400°F. Grease a large rimmed baking sheet with oil.

USING A SHARP KNIFE, cut the squash in half lengthwise (see Tip, opposite). Using a spoon, scoop out the seeds and membranes and discard. Rub 1½ tablespoons of the oil all over the squash halves. Place them cut side down on the prepared baking sheet. Roast until a knife can easily pierce the skin and flesh, 45 to 60 minutes.

IN A SMALL BOWL, whisk together the lime juice, 2 tablespoons of the oil, the honey, 1 teaspoon of the cumin, ½ teaspoon of the salt, and the black pepper. Set aside.

IN A LARGE NONSTICK SKILLET or sauté pan set over medium-high heat, heat the remaining 2 tablespoons oil.

WHEN THE OIL begins to shimmer, add the onion and garlic. Cook, stirring, until slightly soft, about 3 minutes. Add the remaining ½ teaspoon cumin and cook until fragrant, 1 minute. Stir in the bell pepper and black beans, and cook until the bell pepper begins to soften, 2 to 3 minutes. Add the broccoli. Cover and cook until the broccoli is hot, about 5 minutes. Season with the remaining ½ teaspoon salt, and serve.

5½ tablespoons olive oil, plus more for the baking sheet
3 medium acorn squash
3 tablespoons fresh lime juice
2 teaspoons honey
1½ teaspoons ground cumin
1 teaspoon coarse salt
¼ teaspoon freshly ground black pepper
1 small red onion, chopped
2 garlic cloves, chopped
½ medium red bell pepper, chopped
1 (15-ounce) can black beans, rinsed and drained
2 cups frozen broccoli florets

PER SERVING

CALORIES: 230
FAT: 15 g
SODIUM: 1,426.4 mg
CARBOHYDRATE: 23 g
FIBER: 6.1 g
SUGARS: 6.3 g
PROTEIN: 6.5 g

ZUCCHINI
RIBBON "PASTA"
WITH ROASTED CHERRY TOMATOES

SERVES 4

4 cups cherry tomatoes

4 tablespoons olive oil

2 tablespoons balsamic vinegar

1½ teaspoons coarse salt

½ teaspoon freshly ground black pepper

1 pound zucchini

1 pound yellow squash

4 garlic cloves, chopped

2 tablespoons chopped fresh basil

2 tablespoons chopped fresh flat-leaf parsley

Shredded Parmesan cheese (optional)

Available year-round, yellow squash and zucchini are terrific substitutes for pasta. Most athletes never think of them, but they're great! High in vitamin C and low in carbohydrates, these hot-weather vegetables are distinguished by their soft, thin skins and mild sweet flavor. They can be eaten raw, cooked, or somewhere in between, like in this dish. Avoid overcooking the vegetables, as they will release a lot of water and become soft.

PREHEAT THE OVEN to 425°F. Line a rimmed baking sheet with parchment paper.

IN A MEDIUM BOWL, toss the tomatoes with 2 tablespoons of the oil, the vinegar, ½ teaspoon of the salt, and ¼ teaspoon of the pepper. Transfer to the prepared baking sheet. Roast until the tomatoes burst and begin to caramelize, about 20 minutes.

MEANWHILE, using a vegetable peeler (see Tip), shave long strips of zucchini and yellow squash.

IN A LARGE SAUTÉ PAN set over medium-high heat, heat the remaining 2 tablespoons oil. Add the garlic and cook for about 1 minute. Add the ribbons of squash and cook, using tongs to gently toss the squash, until they begin to soften, 2 minutes (do not overcook). Turn off the heat. Add the roasted tomatoes and their juices, the basil, and parsley. Season with the remaining 1 teaspoon salt and ¼ teaspoon pepper. Serve immediately, with Parmesan sprinkled on top (if using).

TIP: For heavy-duty peeling jobs, I prefer Y-shaped peelers over traditional swivel vegetable ones. They offer better control with a wide grip, stay sharp longer, and work for lefties and righties.

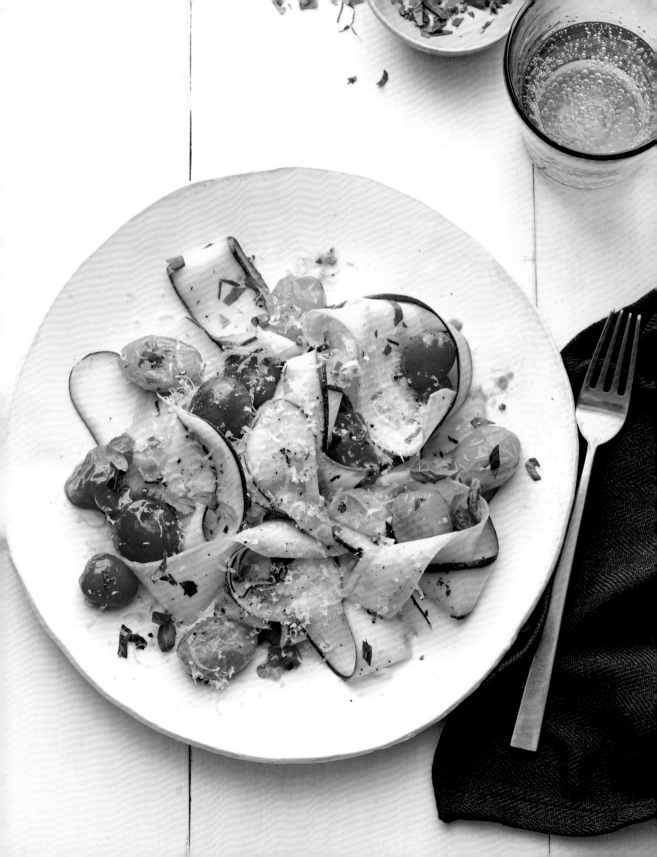

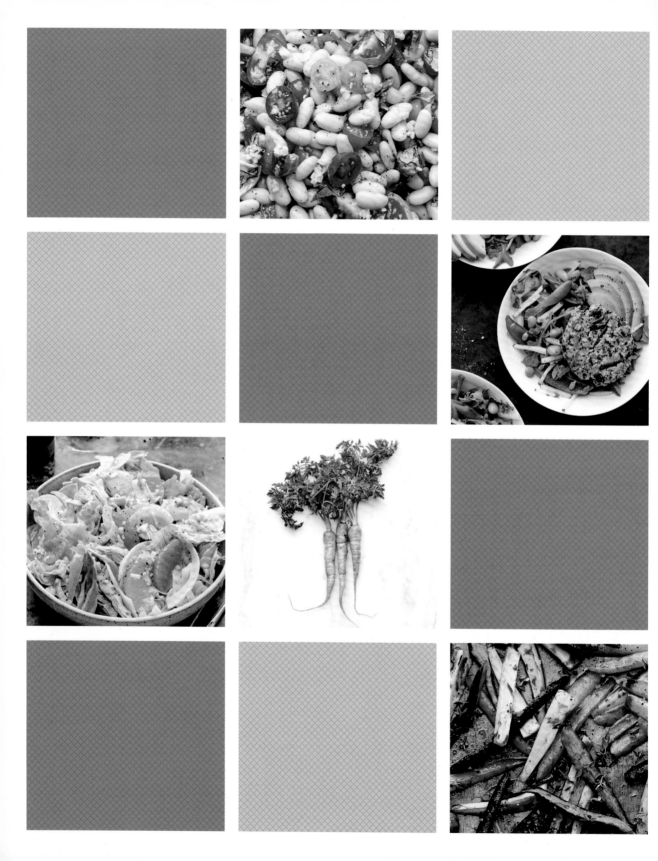

SIDES

SPRING GREEN SALAD

WITH CARROT-GINGER DRESSING

SERVES 4

¾ cup shredded carrot
2 tablespoons chopped onion
2 tablespoons grated or chopped fresh ginger
½ small garlic clove
2 tablespoons rice vinegar
2 tablespoons canola oil
1 tablespoon low-sodium soy sauce
1½ teaspoons honey
3 ounces sugar snap peas
1 (6-ounce) bag baby arugula
1 medium ripe avocado, pitted and diced
½ cup shelled edamame (see Tip)
2 radishes, thinly sliced, for garnish

I love the bright orange dressing that usually comes with salads at Japanese restaurants, but I'm always disappointed with its typical iceberg lettuce blend. I wanted to make a more nutritious and vibrant salad, so I came up with this recipe that features baby arugula, blanched sugar snap peas, omega-3-loaded avocado, and protein-rich edamame. I top off the dish with thin slices of radish for eye-catching color and spicy flavor.

Ginger in particular has great benefits for the athlete, including improving GI problems and acting as an anti-inflammatory, and one study even showed reduced pain response during exercise. So eat up!

IN A BLENDER, combine the carrot, onion, ginger, garlic, vinegar, oil, 2 tablespoons water, the soy sauce, and honey. Blend until smooth. Transfer to a small serving bowl.

BRING A SMALL SAUCEPAN of water to a boil over high heat. Add the sugar snap peas and cook for about 1 minute. Drain immediately and transfer to a bowl of ice water. When cool, drain and pat dry.

ARRANGE THE ARUGULA on a serving platter or on individual serving plates. Scatter the sugar snap peas, avocado, and edamame on top. Garnish with slices of radish. Serve the salad with the dressing on the side.

TIP: Edamame is another name for soybeans. If you're lucky, you can find them fresh, but they're more commonly found frozen in the pod or shelled. Look for them at any supermarket.

SAUTÉED KALE
WITH PEANUT BUTTER SAUCE

SERVES 4

PER SERVING

CALORIES: 98.9
FAT: 7.6 g
SODIUM: 269.7 mg
CARBOHYDRATE: 5.9 g
FIBER: 1.8 g
SUGARS: 1.6 g
PROTEIN: 3.3 g

This recipe was inspired by a friend of mine who made a similar version, which I refined to add a bit of a kick. It can be whipped up in minutes and is delicious served alongside proteins like grilled chicken. To avoid excessive sugar and additives, I prefer to use natural peanut butter. Another key ingredient used here is Liquid Aminos. A gluten-free alternative to soy sauce, Liquid Aminos has a great savory flavor. You can purchase it at health food stores or well-stocked supermarkets.

- 2 tablespoons natural creamy peanut butter, such as Naturally More
- 2 teaspoons Liquid Aminos All Purpose Seasoning or soy sauce
- ¼ cup vegetable broth
- ¼ teaspoon ground coriander
- Pinch of chili powder
- Pinch of ground cumin
- 1 tablespoon toasted sesame oil
- ⅓ yellow onion, chopped
- 1 garlic clove, chopped
- Bunch of kale (see Tip), stems removed, chopped (about 8 ounces)

IN A SMALL BOWL, combine the peanut butter, Liquid Aminos, broth, coriander, chili powder, and cumin. (The mixture should be the consistency of heavy cream. If it's too thick, add more broth or water.) Set aside.

IN A LARGE NONSTICK SAUTÉ PAN set over medium heat, heat the oil. When the oil begins to shimmer, add the onion and garlic and cook, stirring, until soft and translucent, 3 to 5 minutes. Add the kale and cook until the leaves are just wilted, about 3 minutes. Stir in the peanut butter sauce. Toss and serve hot.

TIP: To trim kale stems, place a leaf flat on a cutting board. Using a sharp knife, cut a V-shape around most of the stem to release it from the leaf. Repeat with the other leaves. You can also use this technique for other leafy greens like collards.

TOMATO, BASIL,
AND BEAN SALAD

SERVES 8

- 2 (15-ounce) cans cannellini beans, rinsed and drained
- ½ pound small tomatoes, cut into ½-inch pieces
- ½ cup fresh basil leaves, torn into ½-inch pieces
- 1 teaspoon coarse salt
- ¼ teaspoon freshly ground black pepper
- ¼ cup extra-virgin olive oil
- 4 small garlic cloves, minced

Beans and legumes are great ingredients to have on hand, and you can keep them in your pantry for a long time. Not only are they a source of inexpensive and satisfying protein, they contain low-glycemic-load carbohydrates, fiber, antioxidants, and a host of important vitamins and minerals such as folate, magnesium, iron, and potassium to keep us energized and well fueled. In this salad, I use canned beans for convenience, but I also like to soak beans overnight (dried beans don't have added sodium or other additives; see Tip).

IN A MEDIUM BOWL, combine the beans, tomatoes, basil, salt, and pepper.

IN A SMALL PAN over medium heat, heat the oil. Add the garlic and cook, stirring, until tender, being careful not to let it brown or burn, 1½ to 2 minutes. Pour the garlic and oil over the bean mixture and gently toss. Let stand for 30 minutes before serving.

TIP: To prep dry beans the traditional way, place clean and picked-over beans in a large pot or bowl and cover with 2 inches of water. Let soak overnight. The next day, drain the beans and rinse with cool water. Cover the beans again with 2 inches of cold water, and then bring to a boil over high heat. Reduce the heat to low, cover, and simmer until the beans are tender. Beans can take 30 minutes to 2 hours to cook, depending on the variety.

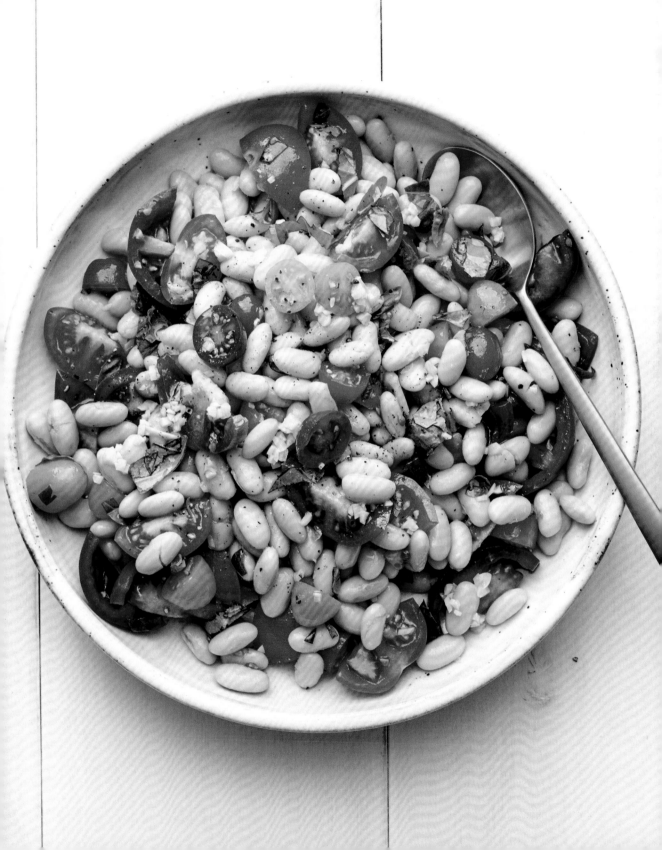

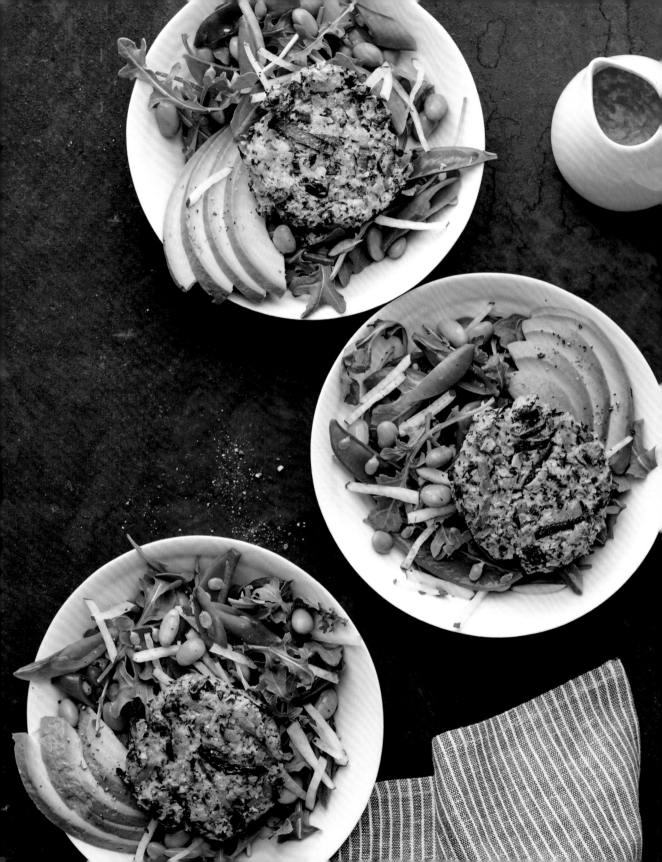

PAN-SEARED
VEGETABLE
PATTIES

MAKES TEN 3- TO 4-INCH PATTIES; SERVES 5

**PER SERVING
(2 PATTIES)**

CALORIES: 40
FAT: 0.5 g
SODIUM: 379.1 mg
CARBOHYDRATE: 6 g
FIBER: 3 g
SUGARS: 1.9 g
PROTEIN: 4.2 g

This quick and easy vegetarian dish can be served as a side or light vegetarian main. As a side, I love it with Turkey-Mozzarella Meat Loaf (page 169) or Quinoa-Crusted Chicken Tenders (page 136). The patties are similar to a vegetable omelet, but without the hefty load of cheese. As an alternative, I pack the silver-dollar-size disks with flavorful herbs that come with little fat, calories, and sodium. I had dried herbs on hand, but you can also use fresh herbs of whatever combination you like. I like to serve these with low-fat sour cream, Sriracha sauce, or ketchup. They're also great served on the Spring Green Salad with Carrot-Ginger Dressing (page 198), as you see in the photo.

1 medium zucchini
1 cup mashed steamed cauliflower
½ cup grated carrot
2 medium scallions (white and green parts), chopped
3 large eggs, beaten
½ teaspoon dried thyme
1 teaspoon dried basil
¾ teaspoon coarse salt
¼ teaspoon freshly ground black pepper
Olive oil cooking spray

USING THE LARGE HOLES OF A BOX GRATER, grate the zucchini. Squeeze the liquid out of the zucchini before measuring 1 cup.

IN A MEDIUM BOWL, combine the zucchini, cauliflower, carrot, scallions, eggs, thyme, basil, salt, and pepper. Stir well.

SPRAY A MEDIUM NONSTICK SKILLET set over medium-high heat with cooking spray. Using a ¼-cup measure, scoop the mixture into the pan 1 inch apart. Cook until browned on one side, 3 to 5 minutes. Flip and cook until cooked through, 2 to 3 minutes. Repeat with the remaining mixture. Serve immediately.

PER SERVING

CALORIES: 169.1
FAT: 4.1 g
SODIUM: 428.5 mg
CARBOHYDRATE: 32.9 g
FIBER: 7.2 g
SUGARS: 11.2 g
PROTEIN: 3.2 g

MASHED
PARSNIPS AND TURNIPS

SERVES 8

- 2½ pounds parsnips, peeled and chopped (see Tip)
- 2 pounds turnips, peeled and chopped
- 12 garlic cloves
- 2 tablespoons extra-virgin olive oil
- 1¼ teaspoons coarse salt
- ½ teaspoon freshly ground black pepper

Cold-weather root vegetables like parsnips and turnips make excellent substitutes for potatoes. When cooked, both vegetables have an earthy, sweet flavor that pairs well with grilled steak or roasted chicken. Have them mashed like in this recipe, or cut them into cubes, toss with some oil, and roast them until browned. I like to serve this with Sage-Rubbed Chicken Breast with Spaghetti Squash (page 139). Any leftovers will keep well; toss them into salads or with quinoa or rice.

PUT THE PARSNIPS, TURNIPS, AND GARLIC in a large saucepan. Cover with water and bring to a boil over medium-high heat. Reduce the heat to low and simmer until tender, about 15 minutes. Drain, reserving about 1 cup of the cooking liquid.

USING A POTATO MASHER, mash the vegetables, adding some of the reserved cooking liquid if it appears too dry. Add the oil and season with the salt and pepper. Serve hot.

TIP: Parsnips are a member of the carrot family and are often mistaken as white carrots. They are quite sweet and have a parsleylike flavor. They can be boiled, roasted, fried, or sautéed.

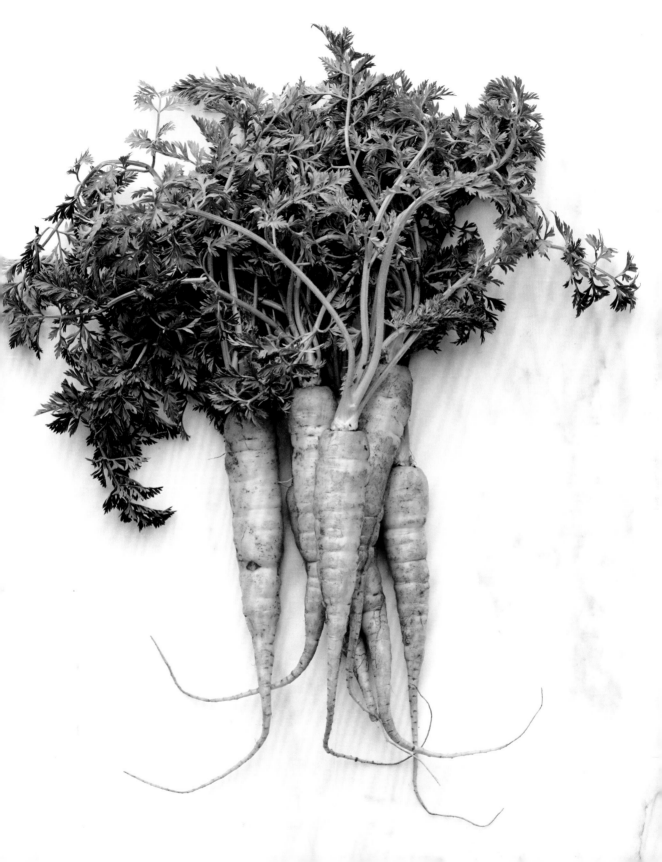

FALAFEL-SPICED
ROASTED CHICKPEAS

MAKES ABOUT 2 CUPS; SERVES 8

1 (29-ounce) can chickpeas, rinsed and drained
¼ cup olive oil
1¼ teaspoons coarse salt
½ teaspoon onion powder
½ teaspoon garlic powder
½ teaspoon ground cumin

Thanks to their impressive nutritional profile—rich in fiber, protein, iron, and complex carbohydrates—it's no wonder chickpeas are having their day in the sun. Here's a snack that I was recently inspired to make after seeing roasted chickpeas for sale in my local supermarket. It's incredibly easy and costs much less than the packaged variety. I also like to make a version substituting sodium-free Italian seasoning for the onion powder, garlic powder, and ground cumin. They're even great with just salt!

PREHEAT THE OVEN to 375°F.

SPREAD OUT THE CHICKPEAS on a rimmed baking sheet lined with paper towels. Shake the chickpeas around and gently pat them dry with more paper towels to remove as much moisture as possible. (The drier the chickpeas, the crispier they will get.)

IN A LARGE BOWL, combine the chickpeas, oil, salt, onion powder, garlic powder, and cumin. Gently stir together until the chickpeas are coated with oil and spices. Divide the mixture between two rimmed baking sheets.

BAKE, shaking the pans every 20 minutes or so, until the chickpeas rattle and are golden, 30 to 40 minutes. Remove the baking sheets from the oven and let cool. The chickpeas will get crispier as they cool.

THE CHICKPEAS will keep in an airtight container for 2 to 3 days.

BALSAMIC MUSHROOMS

MAKES ABOUT 2 CUPS: SERVES 4

PER SERVING

CALORIES: 144
FAT: 13.8 g
SODIUM: 547.2 mg
CARBOHYDRATE: 4.3 g
FIBER: 1 g
SUGARS: 1.6 g
PROTEIN: 2.6 g

This quick and easy recipe can dress up any lean protein or serve as a flavorful addition to salad. I love mushrooms for their rich and earthy flavor, satisfying texture, and versatility in a host of different dishes. They're also great meat substitutes in vegetarian dishes like tacos because of their chewiness and meatlike qualities.

¼ cup olive oil
12 ounces white mushrooms, cleaned and halved (see Tip)
3 tablespoons balsamic vinegar
1 teaspoon coarse salt
¼ teaspoon crushed red pepper flakes
¼ teaspoon freshly ground black pepper

IN A LARGE SKILLET set over medium-high heat, heat the oil. When the oil begins to shimmer, add the mushrooms and cook, stirring, until golden brown, about 5 minutes. Add the vinegar, salt, red pepper flakes, and black pepper. Cook, stirring, for 1 more minute. Serve hot.

TIP: This recipe calls for white mushrooms, but you can substitute others such as portobello or shiitake. To clean, take a damp paper towel and wipe the mushrooms. Never rinse under water. Mushrooms are like sponges and will get waterlogged!

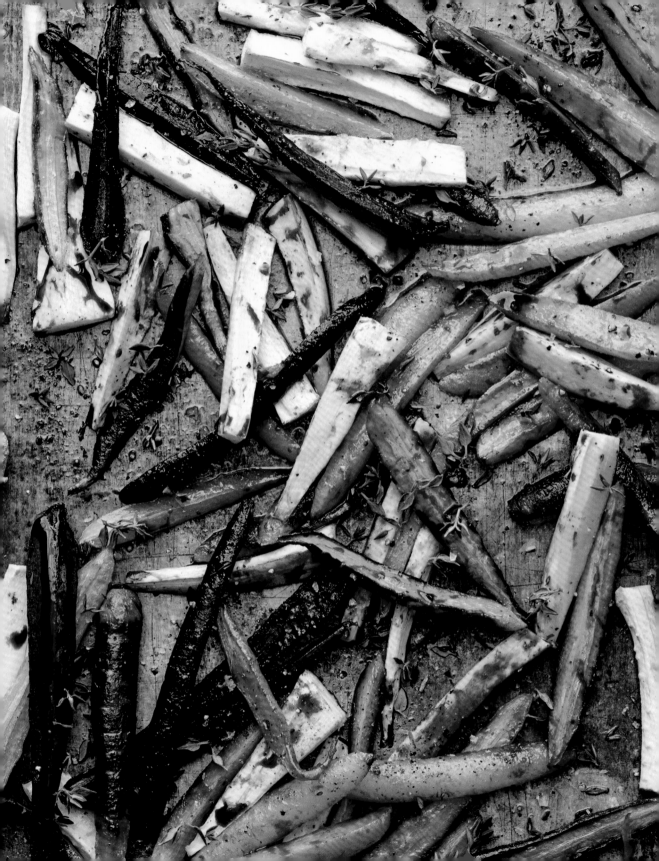

GLAZED
CARROTS AND PARSNIPS

SERVES 6

PER SERVING

CALORIES: 137.9
FAT: 4.9 g
SODIUM: 241.4 mg
CARBOHYDRATE: 23.6 g
FIBER: 4.9 g
SUGARS: 10 g
PROTEIN: 1.8 g

Liven up your fall and winter main dishes with this vegetable side that features naturally sweet carrots and parsnips. When coated with the sweet-and-tart glaze, these root vegetables make a delectable addition to any poultry, meat, fish, or even vegetarian dish. Try them with Salmon Patties over Field Greens (page 140) or Turkey-Mozzarella Meat Loaf (page 169). This side is hearty enough to be its own meal on days when you want something light and vegetarian in nature.

1 pound carrots, peeled and cut into 2-inch sticks
1 pound parsnips, peeled and cut into 2-inch sticks
2 tablespoons olive oil
Leaves from 3 thyme sprigs, roughly chopped (see Tip)
½ teaspoon coarse salt
2 tablespoons balsamic vinegar
1 tablespoon honey

PREHEAT THE OVEN to 375°F.

IN A LARGE BOWL, combine the carrots, parsnips, oil, thyme, and salt. Divide the vegetables between two rimmed baking sheets.

ROAST UNTIL TENDER and lightly browned, about 30 minutes.

MEANWHILE, in a microwave-safe bowl, combine the vinegar and honey. Microwave on high for 15 to 20 seconds. Stir and set aside. After the vegetables have roasted, divide the balsamic-honey mixture between the two pans and toss with the vegetables.

RETURN THE PANS to the oven and roast until the glaze begins to coat the vegetables, 10 more minutes. Serve hot or at room temperature.

TIP: Dried and fresh herbs cannot be substituted on a one-to-one basis, because dried herbs are usually three times as potent as fresh herbs. So if you need 1 teaspoon of dried thyme and only have fresh, multiply by three to get 3 teaspoons (or 1 tablespoon) fresh thyme.

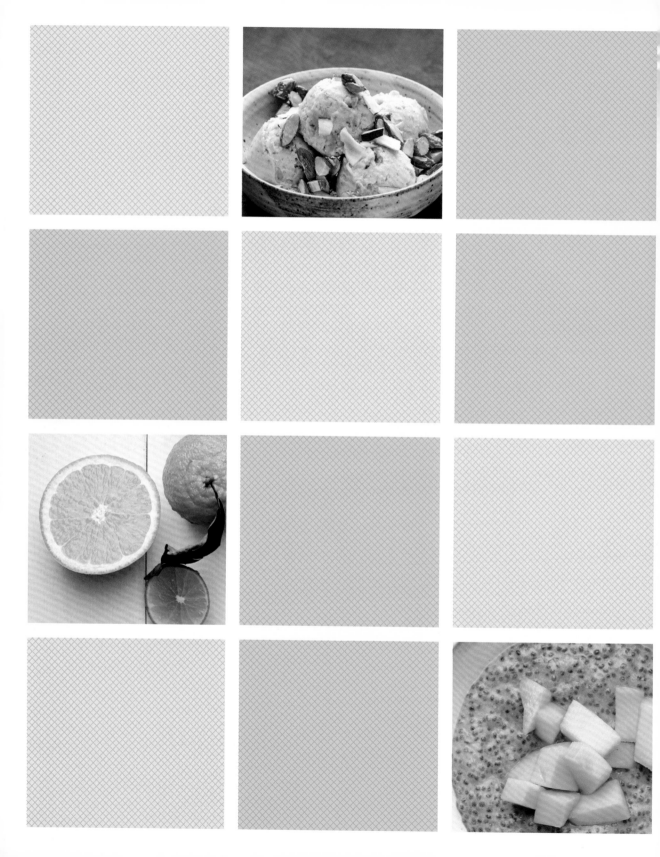

DESSERTS

**MANGO CHIA
PUDDING**

213

**CHOCOLATE
CHIA PUDDING**

214

**SPICED BAKED
APPLES WITH RAISINS
AND WALNUTS**

215

**BANANA "ICE CREAM"
WITH GLAZED ALMONDS
AND TOASTED COCONUT**

216

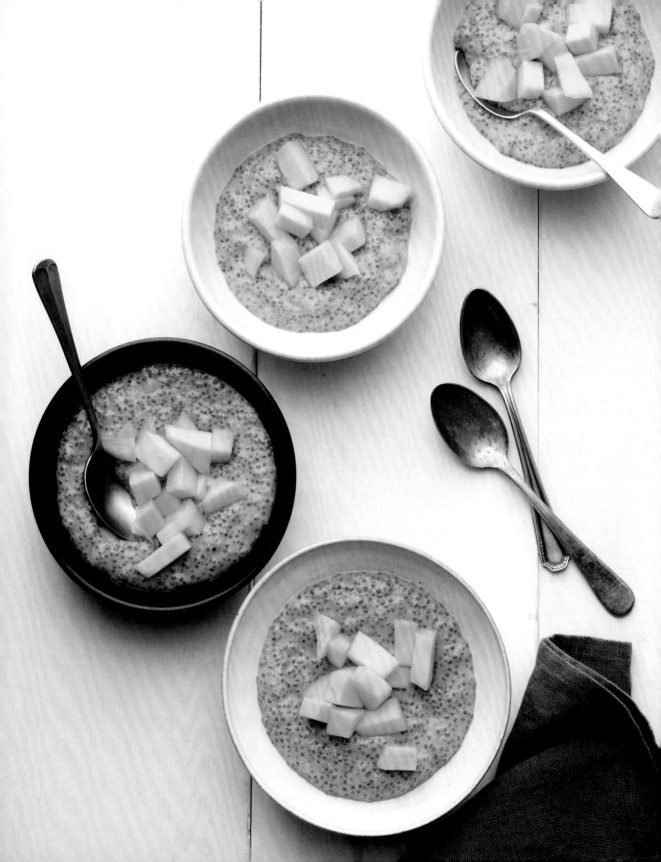

MANGO CHIA PUDDING

SERVES 4

PER SERVING

CALORIES: 201.8
FAT: 11.4 g
SODIUM: 79.8 mg
CARBOHYDRATE: 24.7 g
FIBER: 11.5 g
SUGARS: 12.2 g
PROTEIN: 7 g

While this is definitely a sweet treat, it has no added sugar, and chia seeds are hydration powerhouses. Mangoes, which provide a subtle sweetness here, are a good source of fiber and vitamins A and C. They're also a source of potassium, a mineral that's beneficial for the heart but that we lose through our sweat.

2½ cups unsweetened vanilla coconut milk, plus more as needed the next day
2 cups chopped ripe (see Tip) mango (from 1 large mango)
½ cup chia seeds

IN A BLENDER, blend the coconut milk and 1 cup of the mango until smooth. Transfer to a bowl and stir in the chia seeds. Cover and let set overnight. The next day, add more milk if the mixture is too thick.

TO SERVE, spoon the pudding into each of four serving cups and top with the remaining 1 cup chopped mango.

TIP: A mango is ripe when it gives a little when pressed and gives off a sweet aroma. Mangoes can be stored uncut for up to a week in the refrigerator, or 2 to 3 days cut.

PER SERVING

CALORIES: 185.6
FAT: 9.1 g
SODIUM: 43 mg
CARBOHYDRATE: 27.1 g
FIBER: 11.7 g
SUGARS: 11.8 g
PROTEIN: 6 g

CHOCOLATE CHIA PUDDING

SERVES 6

½ cup chia seeds
(see Tip)
2 cups unsweetened
almond milk
¼ cup unsweetened
cocoa powder
¼ cup honey
½ teaspoon vanilla
extract
2 tablespoons
toasted slivered
or sliced almonds
(see Tip, page 99)
1 pint fresh
raspberries

Rich in omega-3 fatty acids and fiber, chia seeds in recent years have gone from kitschy gift (hello, Chia Pets!) to trendy health food. In terms of the core diet, chia seeds are just that—seeds—and are great to consume anytime during the day between workouts. Chia seeds can be prepared in a variety of ways, but when mixed with liquid, they swell and take on a soft, gelatinous texture that's like tapioca. Here, I've made a dairy-free pudding using chia seeds and the rich flavor of cocoa. I top it with almonds and raspberries, but you could use other toppings, or leave them out—whatever you prefer.

IN A LARGE BOWL OR MASON JAR, whisk or shake together the chia seeds, almond milk, cocoa powder, honey, and vanilla. Cover and refrigerate overnight.

DIVIDE THE PUDDING among six bowls, top with the almonds and raspberries, and serve.

TIP: Health food stores and well-stocked supermarkets will carry chia seeds. Look for them in the grain or specialty food sections. Keep them well sealed in a dry, cool place.

SPICED BAKED APPLES
WITH RAISINS AND WALNUTS
SERVES 8

PER SERVING
CALORIES: 141.9
FAT: 3.5 g
SODIUM: 40.3 mg
CARBOHYDRATE: 22.2 g
FIBER: 2.7 g
SUGARS: 14.9 g
PROTEIN: 6.8 g

Apples contain two types of dietary fiber: soluble and insoluble. Soluble fiber promotes heart health by lowering cholesterol via absorption of bile, and insoluble fiber helps with digestion health by acting as a cleaner as it moves thorough your colon. Outside of nutrition, apples are versatile and just taste great. Just be careful eating them too close to a run, as the fiber content can irritate your stomach.

4 medium Gala apples
1 teaspoon fresh lemon juice
4 teaspoons light butter (see Tip, page 103), at room temperature
¼ teaspoon ground cinnamon
Pinch of ground nutmeg
¼ cup black or golden raisins, chopped
¼ cup chopped walnuts
¾ cup unsweetened apple juice or cider
2 cups nonfat Greek yogurt, such as Fage

PREHEAT THE OVEN to 350°F.

CUT THE APPLES in half and use a melon baller to remove the core and seeds, creating a small cavity for the filling. Place the apples cut side up in a baking dish. Sprinkle the lemon juice over the apples.

IN A SMALL BOWL, combine the butter, cinnamon, nutmeg, raisins, and walnuts. Place heaping teaspoons of the mixture into the center of the apples. Pour the apple juice into the bottom of the dish and cover tightly with foil.

BAKE until the apples are tender but not mushy, about 40 minutes. Remove the foil and bake until the apples are golden, 5 to 10 more minutes.

TO SERVE, dollop each apple half with ¼ cup Greek yogurt.

BANANA "ICE CREAM"
WITH GLAZED ALMONDS AND TOASTED COCONUT

SERVES 2

2 teaspoons honey
Pinch of ground cinnamon
¼ cup roasted unsalted almonds
4 large ripe bananas, cut into small chunks and frozen
2 tablespoons toasted unsweetened coconut (see Tip, page 155)

Bananas, an athlete's best friend, are highly valued for their portability, taste, and nutrition (especially for their potassium). One lesser known use for bananas is to make ice cream! Yes, that's right, you can make a creamy one-ingredient "ice cream" with bananas, and without adding sugar, cream, or eggs. The trick is to cut bananas into small chunks and then freeze them. Once frozen, run them through a homogenizer. For those of you with juicers, many of the auger-style versions also double as a homogenizer, which is perfect for this purpose. If you don't have a homogenizer, blend the chunks in a blender until they begins to resemble ice cream. Just be careful not to overblend, or else you'll end up with banana soup!

PUT THE HONEY in a small microwave-safe bowl. Microwave on high until it is bubbly, 10 to 15 seconds. Stir in the cinnamon.

IN A SMALL NONSTICK SAUTÉ PAN set over medium heat, warm the almonds while constantly shaking the pan. Pour the honey mixture over the almonds and stir to coat. Cook until the nuts are shiny, 1 to 2 minutes. Spread the almonds in a single layer on a greased or parchment-lined plate. Let cool for 10 to 15 minutes. Roughly chop.

PLACE THE BANANAS in a homogenizer, blender, or food processor. Blend until the bananas begin to look smooth and creamy. Scoop the "ice cream" into two bowls and serve with the almonds and toasted coconut sprinkled on top.

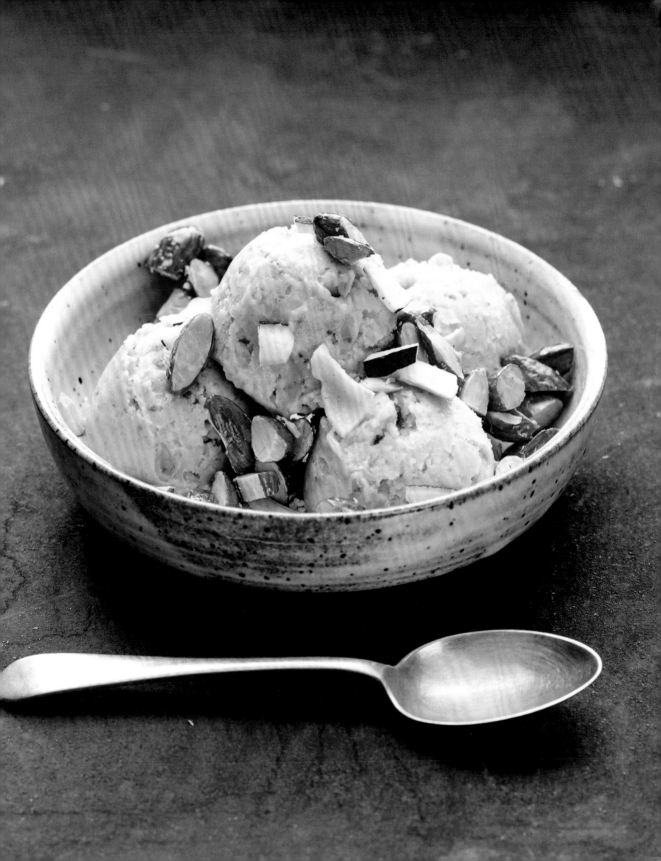

ACKNOWLEDGMENTS

WRITING A BOOK is way more difficult and complex than it sounds! That's what I have learned throughout the process of creating this book. However, there were many folks who made the process a lot easier than it would have been without their help.

First off, none of what I do would be possible without the support of my amazing wife, Chrissie, and our kids, Colin and Stella. Long days and late nights don't happen by themselves, and I'm grateful for my amazing support crew back at home.

To my second family, the Core Diet and QT2 staff, who help support my vision of cutting-edge nutrition and endurance-sports-preparation approaches on a daily basis. These guys and girls work hard because they love what we do, and that passion is what makes the wheels turn and lets us help athletes as well as we are able. Specific thanks to Tim Snow for helping with the actual assembly of this book!

To my third family, the professional athletes I coach; these individuals challenge me to come up with better, more efficient, and cutting-edge nutrition and training approaches every single day. Much of the information in this book was developed as a result of them challenging me daily and my response to deliver real solutions that work.

Thank you to Penguin Random House and specifically my editor, Ashley Meyer, who helped guide me throughout this entire process. She not only created the spark for this book up front, but also helped guide a total novice to create a piece of work that resembles that of a seasoned author. I'm proud of it, Ashley! Thank you! And to the rest of the Harmony Books team: Diana Baroni, Tammy Blake, Sean Civale, Kelley Galbreath, Stephanie Huntwork, Sonia Persad, Patricia Shaw, Kim Tyner, and Aaron Wehner.

Although the concepts in this book are ones I've developed over many years, I had the privilege of working with Shirley Fan to bring them to life. Her dynamic and fresh recipes do just that, and tasting many of her dishes during the photo shoot for the book really had me excited to get this book into the hands of athletes.

Last, I want to thank the athletes featured in the photos of the book: Linsey Corbin, Pedro Gomes, Dan Moore, and Caitlin Snow. Thank you for being part of this project!

INDEX

ABOUT THE AUTHOR

JESSE KROPELNICKI is a veteran professional triathlon coach and the founder of QT2 Systems brand of endurance sports preparation businesses, which includes QT2 Systems, the Core Diet, OutRival Racing, and the Run Formula. His roster of clients includes IRONMAN champions and past USAT national team athletes. He lives with his wife and their two kids in Scituate, Massachusetts.